Assessment of clinical practice:
The why, who, when and how of assessing nursing practice

Assessment of clinical practice:
The why, who, when and how of assessing nursing practice

by

Jane Walton and Maggie Reeves

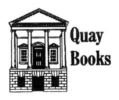

Quay
Books

£ 17.78

Quay Books Division, Mark Allen Publishing Ltd
Jesses Farm, Snow Hill, Dinton, Wiltshire, SP3 5HN

British Library Cataloguing-in-Publication Data
A catalogue record is available for this book

© Mark Allen Publishing Ltd 1999
Reprinted 2001
ISBN 1 85642 084 1

Reprinted in the UK by IBT Global, London

Contents

Acknowledgements

This book is written for all those involved in the assessment of nursing staff. It is written as a result of the many situations that the authors and their colleagues have found themselves in while assessing students, and from the questions that students and potential assessors have raised.

We would like to thank those people who have encouraged and supported the writing of this book, in particular Hilary Walker for her guidance and for writing the foreword and Dr Helen Barrett for giving the time to read the ongoing work.

Special thanks also to David Walton and Mike Reeves for their continued support and help.

Preface

The why, who, when and how of assessing nursing practice. This book presents a way by which assessment in nursing practice can be looked at critically to determine safe practice by both assessor and assessee.

Everything about assessment has a meaning. It questions our perception, our values, our beliefs, our knowledge, our memory, our standards and it can give us guidance, motivation, rewards and hopefully confidence. This confidence should encourage the maintenance of competent practice in order to promote excellence in care delivery. The format of this book includes information, with selected scenarios and guided activities, to enable critical appraisal of assessment.

The overall purpose of the book is to encourage the reader to think about and analyse his or her own standards, expectations, observations and interpretations of nursing practice.

This book is aimed at anyone involved in the assessment of clinical practice, with or without a formal assessment qualification. It includes the assessment of qualified nurses, student nurses and those undertaking an NVQ training.

This book cannot guarantee to give you undisputed answers but it is hoped that it will make you think and question not only assessment, but also the practice of nursing.

It must be said that assessment can be fraught with problems — take a minute to think whether there is a qualified nurse that you know who you would not be happy to have nursing you.

If there is such a person then the assessment of that nurse is likely to have been inadequate.

What could have been done? Read on.

Foreword

The last two years have seen major changes in the assessment of the knowledge, skills and attitudes of students undertaking preparation to enter the Professional Register for Nurses, Midwives and Health Visitors. An increasing emphasis has been placed on the value of learning undertaken in the clinical environment and its credit worthiness. This shift in the formal recognition of work-based learning is requiring assessors to develop new knowledge, skills and attitudes that enable the accurate measuring and recording of experiential learning.

Teaching assessors to assess constructively requires a professional attitude which involves devoting time and commitment to the process. Thorough learning of the strategies to be used is an essential tool for this process.

This book will be a valuable learning tool for both assessor and assessee. It logically examines the process of theory of assessment before progressing onto the practice, allowing the reader to reflect on the process through the provision of structured exercises and examples of the way in which decisions can be made and verified.

The use of two students who exhibit differing attitudes to assessment give the text a feeling of reality and will stimulate the assessor to introduce impartiality to the process while considering the development of individual personalities within the context of professional outcomes.

HJ Walker
Education officer
English National Board for Nursing,
Midwifery and Health Visiting
July 1998

How to use this book

This book contains activities and scenarios. These are intended to complement the content.

The activities are for the reader to undertake at the specified intervals. They are strongly recommended but are not essential to the understanding of the chapter. They may also be used as discussion points.

The scenarios are used to illustrate and place in reality the points being made. They can also be used as discussion points.

In some scenarios names will be used for two students under discussion. Their names are Jessica Jeopardy and Danny Danger.

The following terms will be used throughout the book:

The assessor will be known as she and nurse will be known as s/he.

The patient will be known as he.

The student or learner in the assessment situation will mostly be referred to as assessee. In some instances the term learner will be used to refer to both student and learner, both pre- and post-registration.

The term assistant will be used for the health care assistants in the instance of National Vocational Qualification (NVQ) discussion.

The two students referred to in this book are Jessica and Danny:

* **Jessica** has wanted to be a nurse for as long as she can remember. Academically she is very bright and can often put forward a theoretical argument with assertive, logical presentation. Practically she is more timid and likes a well-reasoned argument for each action. This approach to the work in clinical areas often leads to her hanging back and waiting to be asked to complete a task. Once asked, she often wants a full justification of how and why it is done that way. She feels that she is often working without adequate reason or explanation of the work.

* **Danny** went to university after leaving school and obtained a third class degree in psychology. The only job he was able to get on leaving university was in a bank. He found working in the bank restrictive due to the hours and the routine of the work was rather

confining. He says he is rather a free spirit and likes work in which he can use his initiative and adaptability to respond. Nursing seems to suit him and he is hoping for a post as a charge nurse or unit manager as soon as he can. He is very friendly and outgoing. He sees nursing as having a good social basis. He finds himself often burning the candle at both ends but feels that he is quite competent at managing his nursing work. Academically, on his nursing course, he is very borderline, and does not seem to put much work into his studies at present.

Introduction

Assessment has many components and interpretations. It is popular with some and provokes anxiety in others. It is widely used in nursing both as a means of determining patients' conditions and their needs and as a measurement of staff achievement.

There are many differing types of assessment. This book will draw examples of assessment from many quarters. It is intended that, although the example may not be of a clinical nature, the principle can be applied to the assessment of practice.

This book will also look at various aspects in relation to the assessment of nursing staff of all specialities and status in the clinical areas.

1

Principles of assessment

Definitions and interpretations of assessment

In order to discuss the definitions and interpretations of assessment the notion of assessment requires exploration.

The variety of words that link to the term assessment help to illustrate the breadth of assessment and how easy it is to differ in opinion.

A full definition of the term and use of assessment can be found in the work of Rowntree (1987):

Assessment occurs whenever one person in some kind of interaction, direct or indirect, with another is conscious of obtaining and interpreting information about the knowledge and understanding or abilities and attitudes of this other person.

Activity 1

Underline the key points of this definition and consider the implication for an assessor.

Examining the key points of this definition highlights some relevant aspects concerning assessment.

* One aspect is the **subjective influence of assessment**. The assessor needs to identify her own subjective influence and render it as objective as possible. One way to do this is through the use of a reliable assessment tool.

* The definition also indicates an important aspect of assessment from the point of view of nursing practice — that is 'the kind of interaction' for assessment of nursing action, this must be 'direct interaction' meaning that what is assessed **must be seen and heard**. In other words, actual occurrences or omissions must be recorded. This is a means of making the assessment more objective. 'Seeing' and 'hearing' raise problems for assessment.

* Another aspect is the obtaining and interpreting of information. This raises the questions of **what** is looked for, **how** and **when**.The aspects of what, how and when are all potential and/or continual problems of assessment.

1

Problems in assessment

Problems vary from:
- how much time should be spent working with the person being assessed?
- can the word of someone else be taken with regard to the performance of a member of staff?
- does an assessor see and hear everything?
- what information does the assessor look for and how is the information interpreted?

How much time an assessor should spend working with a student raises the question of whether an assessor needs to work with a student prior to the assessment. See *chapter 3* for a discussion on mentor and assessor.

Can the word of someone else be taken with regard to the performance of a member of staff?

Activity 2

> Try and describe, to another member of staff, an incident that has happened at work and then ask her to recount the incident to someone else.

Now think about the description given:
- did she explain the same incident?
- did she add or miss any aspects?
- did she put a different emphasis on the information?

If the incident is not similar then questions can be raised as to whether another person can assess and pass on information. It also raises questions concerning memory and perception. Memory and perception can initially affect the assessor, but they can also doubly affect the conveyance of information from one person to another.

Does an assessor see and hear everything? Look at the following situation.

Scenario 1

This incident involves the assessment of a teaching session by two assessors. The aim of the teaching session was to introduce the students to the making of infant feeds. The teacher while making up the feed in front of the students was questioned by the students. The teacher had stated that she was making a collective feed and that she had to put nine scoops into the solution. At the end of the teaching session the teacher's performance was discussed. The discussion revealed the following:

Assessor A had not counted the number of scoops placed into the baby feed.

Assessor B had counted 11 scoops put into the feed.

The teacher herself was unsure of the number due to the fact that a student had questioned her at the time.

What should have been the result of the assessment? See *chapter 6*, page 65, for the role of the assessor.

What does the assessor look for? See *chapter 5*.

In further discussing the principles of assessment the following mnemonic is used based on the word assessment.

Achievable
    Structured
        Seeable
            Educational
                Subjective
                    Selective
                        Measurable
                            Evaluative
                                Notable
                                    Testable

A = Achievable

Unrealistic expectations can discourage ability. For example, the lady who has suffered a stroke and who is told by the nurse that she can go home when she is able to dress herself, before she can even move her right arm.

S = Structured

This aspect should benefit both the assessee and the assessor. Both need to know the assessment expectations from the point of view of performance and outcome. If the assessee does not know what is expected, how can s/he do well? If the assessor does not know what to look for she may look at the wrong aspects.

This could lead to assessment by chance or instances of luck.

S = Seeable

If you do not see an action, how do you know if it was done correctly or if it was done at all?

The following incident occurred in a busy accident and emergency department.

Scenario 2

An infant, who had had a febrile convulsion, was brought in by his mother. The infant was taken into a cubicle and a rectal temperature was taken by a student. A member of staff looked into the cubicle during the temperature taking and noted that the student had placed the thermometer into the rectum the wrong way round. A temperature would have been recorded by the student in the first instance but it would have been an incorrect temperature if the action had not been seen.

This illustrates the point that direct assessment means 'to see'.

E = Educational

Apart from assessing what staff have learnt, assessment is a form of helping them to learn and develop. Assessment covers a wide remit. It is also important to remember that assessment includes three vital components of learning; knowledge, attitudes and skills (Bloom, 1956).

S = Subjective

This is a problem in any type of assessment. Objectivity is the opposite of subjectivity and is an approach to be fostered in assessment. For example, consider the following scenario.

Scenario 3

A friend asks you for your opinion (assessment) of the room which has just been redecorated. It is totally opposite to the type of decoration you would choose. You could reply: a) how awful; b) don't the colours go well with your furniture; c) what a professional finish; d) it looks cleaner and fresher; e) it's quite different from before.
Now consider which of the above statements are subjective and which are objective.

Before the objectivity or subjectivity of these statements is reviewed there is another situation to consider with subjectivity and that concerns the accuracy of the reply.

Consider the following situations:
i)   Your friend has just laughingly put an unsuitable wig on her head and asks your opinion.

ii)   Your friend has recently commenced cytotoxic therapy and has been given the same wig as mentioned in case i) and asks your opinion.

In giving your opinion in the above situations how much of your response will reflect what you think your friend wants to hear? It is questionable whether subjectivity will give the accurate response in all instances. As an assessor the awareness of the result the student wants could influence the feedback of the assessor, without considering the aspect of assessor subjectivity. To avoid both these issues objectivity needs to be achieved. This can be done by giving an accurate statement of your feelings irrespective of your friend's wishes.

Objective statements need to be made.

These are statements of fact as occurred in item d) and e) above; whereas items a), b), and c) are statements of opinion and are therefore subjective. It is worth remembering that productive relationships are produced when communication is constructive, sensitive and honest (Sutherland, 1995).

S = Selective

What needs to be assessed must be assessed. This has a link with the term validity, which is discussed in more detail in *chapter 5*.

Assessment should be able to determine aspects of knowledge, skills and/or attitudes but it cannot assess everything at one time. Nor can too much be included in any one assessment situation.

Take,for example, the situation of a pub meal.

Scenario 4

You are being assessed on your memory of the menus that are displayed on the blackboard by the bar. How many items can you be expected to remember? Try it. If you cannot remember all of them, what about recalling just the main meals and not the desserts as well? After all, you do not always have to order all at the same time.

M = Measurable

Two questions can be posed here:

What is being measured and **how** is it being measured?

Those new to assessment often assume that there must be black and white answers to each problem, for example, a pass or fail. With time and experience it usually becomes clear that this is rather too simplistic a view and that assessment decisions are far more complex.

Think about this situation.

Scenario 5

When cooking are you always sure that you have put the right ingredients in? For example, were 4 or 5 teaspoons put in the mix when the phone rang? Is there a possibility that you lost count of the number of teaspoons used?

A measurement of a teaspoon is easy to identify with but what about the measurement of a professional attitude?

E = Evaluative

This component looks further than the expected outcome; it looks at the validity of the assessment and the results of the assessment, for example, why was there such a poor pass rate on a written test last week? Questions could be asked which might concern the suitability of the assessment, the preparation of the assessees or previous performance of the assessees.

The assessment criteria and the teaching should also come under scrutiny.

N = Notable

Assessment must reflect a noteworthy intent and have a notable purpose. The reason for assessment must be apparent to both the assessor and the assessee. The timing, type and content of assessment must all be relevant to the intent.

Assessment is not intended to make life stressful by creating a series of hurdles for people to jump. Hurdles such as assignments, oral examinations, practical demonstrations and unseen written examinations must have a valid reason in the assessment of learning.

A notable aspect of learning is that learning should be permanent but this is questionable.

Consider the following situations:

Scenario 6

Driving a car — How many of you who drive, do so as you did when you passed your test? Are you a safe driver now? Think of what will happen if the proposal for 5-yearly driving tests becomes a reality.

Scenario 7

Handwashing — Poor hand hygiene is said to be a main cause of the spread of infection. A nurse may be assessed on his/her handwashing technique, but how many nurses persist with that same practice of safe handwashing following instruction and assessment?

Research has shown poor standards of handwashing techniques (Elliot 1996, Taylor, 1978).

T = Testable

Assessment must measure the assessee, the teacher and the form of instruction being followed. It should indicate whether there is satisfactory performance. In nursing it is important that performance is safe at the time of assessment. This safe action at assessment should help to maintain a satisfactory standard of performance.

However, this raises the question of whether a satisfactory standard of performance at the time of assessment really does guarantee a consistent safe performance. It is questionable as to when assessment testing should occur but also whether the testing does produce a learnt behaviour or whether continual testing is required.

According to the *Collins English Dictionary* (1984) to assess means to determine, estimate or judge — but in nursing what are we assessing?

Roget's Thesaurus (1987) lists the following words linked to the word assess: measure, estimate, and appraise.

Neither of these definitions actually includes two of the key terms of assessment, those of validity and reliability. These will be discussed later, on *pages 43 and 44.*

It is stated by Rowntree (1987) that assessment is 'awash with hidden assumptions, unstated values, partial truths, confusion of ideas, false distinctions and irrelevant emphases'.

This poses the question of **why** assessment is undertaken.The following chapter will address this issue.

Conclusion

At the end of this chapter the reader should be able to:
- define the term assessment
- list six words that have a meaning in assessment
- identify three key problems with assessment
- consider responses to the following situations (refer back to *pages xiii–xiv* for personality profiles of Jessica and Danny):
  * Jessica asks you in her normal timid fashion to justify the reason for her having to be assessed in your particular area when she is only there for ten shifts.
  * Danny confidently says that he is only there to observe so why should he need any assessment as surely he should be assessing the staff he is observing.

References and further reading related to this section

Bloom B (1956) *Taxonomy of Educational Objectives: The Classification of Educational Goals. Handbook One: Cognitive Domain.* McKay, New York

Hanks P, ed (1984) *Collins Dictionary of English Language.* Collins, London and Glasgow

Cotton J (1995) *The Theory of Assessment — An Introduction.* Kogan Page, London

Elliott PRA (1996) Handwashing practice in nurse education. *Prof Nurse* **11**(6): 357–360

Quinn FM (1995) *Principles and Practice of Nurse Education,* 3rd edn. Chapman Hall, London

Kirkpatrick B, ed (1987) *Roget's Thesaurus of English Words and Phrases.* Cox & Wyman, Reading

Rowntree D (1987) *Assessing Students: How shall we know them?* Kogan Page, London

Sutherland JA (1995) The Johari Window: A strategy for teaching therapeutic confrontation. *Nurse Educ* **20** (3): 22–24

Taylor LJ (1978) An evaluation of handwashing techniques — 1. *Nurs Times* Jan 12: 54–55

Taylor LJ (1978) An evaluation of handwashing techniques — 2. *Nurs Times* Jan 19: 108–110

2
Why assess?

Activity 3

Before reading this chapter, list as many reasons as you can for having assessment within the education of nurses.

Please note that Klug (1974) has actually identified 32 reasons for assessment. Your list might not be as comprehensive.

A broad statement of the reasons for assessment comes from Quinn (1995), who argues that it benefits the student, the teacher and other people. In nursing the 'other people' could be the patients.

Assessment therefore is seen as forming an important component of the nursing curriculum and professional preparation.

Rowntree (1987) summarises the need for assessment within the following:

i)   selection process
ii)   maintenance of standards
iii) motivation of students
iv)   feedback to students
v)   feedback to the teacher
vi)   preparation for life.

This chapter will now look at each reason in turn. You will need to reflect on your current knowledge; you might find it useful to document your thoughts.

i) Selection process

Activity 4

Think about the following:
What were the selection criteria used to select you for your current position?
Consider the criteria on the application form and at the interview.
List some of the questions you were asked on the application form and at the interview and consider why these may have been asked.
Discuss with a colleague whether you found the interview easy or difficult and why.

To start you thinking, this section will look at a few typical interview questions and indicate the rationale, or in assessment terms, the validity of the questions.

Assessment during interview

Question   'Why have you applied for this job?'

Rationale   Assessment of interest and/or motivation for the job.

Question   'What can you offer the job?'

Rationale   Assessment of your potential from the point of view of the employer.

Question   'Why should you have the job instead of the other candidates?'

Rationale   Assessment of your particular skills, eg. assertiveness and enthusiasm.

Question   'What are your weaknesses?'

Rationale   Assessment of your self-image and your needs for development, plus your suitability for the job.

As in all assessments the questions asked must have some relevance to the situation: in other words, there must be a **valid** reason for asking the questions and there must be a reliable decision made on the basis of the answers.

Not only does the assessor have to ask the right questions but also the right method of assessment should be selected to match the intended outcome.

Brown (1997) suggests that assessment needs to be more innovative and possibly new methods need to be adopted.

Interviewing applicants for nurse education and for job appointments has been subjected to various methods of assessment including analysis of handwriting, psychometric testing or profiling. No method has proved infallible; therefore, one answer is that a selection of methods may be needed.

Activity 5

> Think about whether you feel it is important to have a selection process for entry to the nursing profession: a) as a student and b) as a qualified nurse.
> If you feel that there should be a selection process can you suggest and justify a means?

It would seem that there does need to be some form of selection for entry onto the register for nurses at the completion of the training/

education course. The question of whether nursing is a profession has been debated for a long time. One criterion for a profession is a selective entry both to training/education and to subsequent entry to the profession (Lorentzon, 1992).

One reason for the selection of a person for a profession is related to the position and the expectations of society. These expectations can be linked to the work to be performed and the related expected standard.

ii) Maintenance of standards

What is a standard?

A standard, according to the College of Occupational Therapists (1989–1991) is:

> *an acceptable or approved example or statement of something against which measurement and/or judgement takes place; a level of quality relevant to the activity.*

Standards and standard setting have been 'buzz words' over the last decade. In the clinical context actions are measured against 'standard statements' which include criteria for determining whether or not the standard has been met.

Examples of standards

* The patient's name and unit number must be shown on every piece of nursing documentation.

* The patient's pressure sore risk must be documented within two hours of admission and, thereafter, weekly until discharge.

* The patient's care plan must contain the patient's nursing needs, an achievable goal and the required nursing care.

* Each student nurse must have an initial interview with his/her mentor within six hours of being on the clinical placement.

Activity 6

Think about the following:
What four standards can you identify that you attempt to achieve in your clinical area?
How do you know that you have achieved the standards set?

The standards that you have set for yourself are most probably the 'desired and achievable levels of performance against which actual practice is compared' (Quinn, 1995). They are standards that may conform to the clinical practice guidelines for your area and will reflect the special needs of your patients/clients or practice area. One of the associated standard statements for your clinical area might be the way staff communicate in a friendly, informative manner when answering the telephone. The member of staff will state the ward title, own name and ask, 'how may I help you?'

For further information on standards and assessment see *chapter 5* on tools for assessment.

iii) Motivation of students

Assessment may motivate students to respond and demonstrate their learning. This motivation may occur as a result of impending assessment or it may come from the assessor's response to the assessee's performance during assessment or it may come from the assessment result. Whatever the motivating force, motivation is seen as a key component related to learning.

This section will look at some aspects of motivation and link them to performance and assessment. This will involve the reader in some personal reflection as well as giving some indication for future performance, especially as an assessor.

Before reading further on motivation you may like to carry out the following activity.

Activity 7

Write down what the term motivation means to you and what motivates you to want to learn and work.

Much has been written about motivation; only a small range of aspects will be discussed here.

Theories and definitions of motivation attempt to explain the reasons why people behave in one way rather than another.

According to Child (1986), a person is motivated by an internal process. The resultant motivation is to satisfy this internal process be it physical or psychological. This internal process can be described as a drive or need. Drives which motivate people to satisfy particular needs for themselves, such as hunger, are known as intrinsic factors.

Maslow (1971) classifies 'needs' in a hierarchy and argues that higher level needs cannot be addressed if lower level needs are not satisfied and achieved.

Maslow's hierarchy of needs

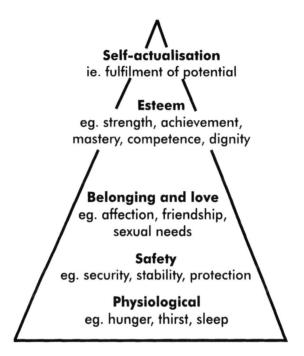

Self-actualisation
ie. fulfilment of potential

Esteem
eg. strength, achievement,
mastery, competence, dignity

Belonging and love
eg. affection, friendship,
sexual needs

Safety
eg. security, stability, protection

Physiological
eg. hunger, thirst, sleep

Activity 8

It is worth thinking about whether motivation theory may explain:
- why some people are keen to learn while others are not?
- why some people do well while others do not
- whether motivating people adequately would achieve better assessment results.

What are your opinions? Consider the following:
- does assessment actually motivate people to learn
- do people learn only the information for the assessment?

McClelland *et al* (1953) discuss motivation as linked to achievement. They propose that some people have an intrinsic need for achievement which motivates them to grow and develop. Achieving well is important to these people and assessment feedback can indicate how well they have achieved.

This recognition of achievement could justify the need for and importance of assessment. Assessment can identify levels of achievement, mastery and/or competence. All these levels of achievement can be recognised within Maslow's hierarchy.

Studies (McClelland *et al,* 1953) have shown that people with a high level of need to achieve do better on tests and problem solving and mathematics. So some people may thrive on assessment while others may be motivated to learn for other reasons. According to Weiner (1979), an individual's need for understanding may in itself be an important reason for behaviour/learning which may be unrelated to any assessment. Examples of this may be found in hobbies: a person tries to understand how to play cards not because they are being assessed but because of a need to improve understanding or a need to enjoy a competition, or a gamble. Other examples could include the need to learn swimming as an interest or for self-preservation.

Intrinsic factors can also be disincentives to learn, especially if the person gets very nervous about doing well. This may be the case with a mature student who has returned to college after a long absence and then feels anxious about his/her abilities.

There are also external influences (extrinsic factors) that will influence behaviour and make people act in certain ways: these include incentives or rewards such as praise. Extrinsic factors come from outside the person and take their meaning from the particular social context within which they occur, eg. a box of toffees to a child for doing well at school as compared to a box of toffees given to a nurse on achieving his/her registration. The reward must be appropriate, otherwise it can lead to demotivation.

Consider the situation of an assessor who is always known to reward the student with a pass grade regardless of the student's performance. This may lead to a reduced, demotivated performance by a student who realises that s/he does not have to perform at his/her best to achieve a pass.

Activity 9

Refer back to *activity 7* and see if you can identify whether your reasons for wanting to learn and work were intrinsic or extrinsic reasons, or a mixture of both.

Whatever the motivation, students need feedback regarding achievement.

iv) Feedback to students

Feedback needs to be both relevant and useful. If a student perceives the comments to be irrelevant and/or unworkable, the comments will

be ignored. Ignored comments will not assist in motivating the student to perform.

Activity 10

> List three examples of intrinsic and extrinsic factors that affect how hard you work in your clinical area.

While assessing a student it is not possible to know about the differing motivational forces. However, the possibility that what an assessor says can be either motivating or demotivating must always be considered. Feedback can provide extrinsic rewards, which may in turn lead to increased enthusiasm for engaging in the learning process (ie. intrinsic reward). Intrinsic factors may be a personal sense of perfectionism or the desire to please another; this could mean pleasing the assessor or the patient.

Intrinsic motivation is considered a more valuable force for learning as the student will search out and learn from self-motivation. Self-motivation is considered to be the means by which adult learners learn more effectively (Knowles, 1984).

Consider the following feedback (verbal responses of acknowledgement) made by an assessor to the assessee:

'Good, you have done that very well.'

'Good, you have completed that well, but possibly you could include this also.'

'You have completed that task adequately but there are several areas which require improvement.'

'Why did you do it like that?'

'I see that you have done that but it is incorrect.'

'Stop! You are doing that all wrong.'

Each of these statements, if said during or after performing an action, would have an effect on the assessee. The more positive comments are liable to have a positive effect on his/her motivation and spur him/her on, whereas the negative comments may spur him/her on but possibly not with such a positive frame of mind.

Absence of feedback is always likely to demotivate. Very little can be learnt from silence which can indicate to the student anything from acceptable performance on his/her part to lack of interest and/or rejection on the part of the assessor.

It is **not** a case of 'no news is good news'.

Activity 11

> List five occasions when it was possible to give feedback
> (acknowledgement) to students/staff in your clinical area.
> Choose one example and describe how feedback was given.

Acknowledgement of, and comments about, performance may be perceived by the recipient in a positive or negative way.

A major aim of feedback is that any criticism should be constructive and perceived as such.

Constructive criticism

Activity 12

> Explain in your own words your understanding of the term
> constructive criticism. Give an example of constructive criticism.

Many people see constructive criticism as finding fault; it should not be viewed in this way. Criticism can be of several types:

- making an unfavourable or severe judgement or comment. This can appear destructive.
- evaluating or analysing work. This could be seen as either destructive or constructive.

Constructive can mean serving to build or improve.

Constructive criticism therefore needs to be seen as:

- a positive analysis that serves to improve behaviour.

Assessment feedback is used to report on a person's performance to help personal development. It is said that we are never too old to learn, so in assessment of performance there may always be the possibility of development — something that can be learnt from the situation.

There may also be the need for correction but this should be handled in the positive light of constructive criticism. No one likes to be told that they are wrong but they can be told of corrective or improved behaviour in a positive way.

For example:

You have completed that task competently in the time stipulated but possibly you need to pay some more attention to communication with the patient during the procedure. How do you think this could be done?

This sort of constructive criticism incorporates the fact that assessment should be a two way process: that is, assessment by self or another. It also takes into account the need to enjoy learning and to feel positive about one's ability to learn. In other words, it provides intrinsic motivation and, in Maslow's scheme of things, this satisfies needs at several levels, eg. need for safety (to make mistakes and learn), need for esteem (recognition), belonging (acceptance), need for self-actualisation (recognising one's full potential).

Activity 13

Think of some examples of feedback to students that you have experienced by both giving and receiving. By completing the following chart, list the advantages and disadvantages:

	Positive feedback	Negative feedback
As assessor		
As assessee		

v) Feedback to the teacher/first level nurse

The term 'teacher' here is used loosely to indicate any nurse involved in assisting the process of learning in another.

In reflecting on the value of feedback for a teacher it can be seen that feedback from students can be a form of assessment of the teacher.

This can be done formally by the use of evaluation forms or informally 'via the grapevine', ie. the comments made in a break period or between students after a teaching session that get reported back to the teacher via another source. The principles of constructive criticism are important here too.

Assessment from the teacher's perspective

Assessment can be a demotivator for the teacher. As a teacher you may have taught a subject, felt that it went well and then the students do not do well in a test, or, you overhear the students saying, 'Oh that was so boring'.

A teacher cannot get it right for everyone all of the time, but then neither do all students enjoy the same sessions for a whole assortment of reasons. Also, it is fair to say that all students do not learn in the same way or at the same rate.

Assessment does not come in the right way or at the right time for all students. Some students may prefer practical work with little theoretical input: the 'activists' according to Honey and Mumford (1986). Other students might like a written test rather than a practical test as this allows them to demonstrate their wide reading and their ability to analyse an issue critically: the 'theorists', as described by Honey and Mumford (1986). The reflectors and the pragmatists in the Honey and Mumford model would prefer other types of assessment, such as a reflective journal or a feasibility study.

Assessing, like teaching, needs to be dynamic. It can help teachers to:

- make sure that they are assisting the students to learn in the best way
- measure the attainment of students
- identify problem areas in the nursing programme
- learn and develop their own approach to the teaching/learning dyad.

Overall, to improve assessment it is important to balance feedback from self and others. For a variety of reasons some people can be too harsh or too lenient when assessing themselves and/or others.

vi) Preparation for life

There are a multitude of assessments that a person will be subjected to both at work and at play. In the working career of nurses, assessment will come from patients, clients, peers, colleagues, senior staff, managers, relatives, family, tutorial staff and even self. The means of these assessments will vary.

Activity 14

Make a list of the variety of ways by which you have been assessed throughout your life. Look at the assessments linked to your work and identify who assessed you.

Means of assessment

There are many different means of assessment including examinations (seen and unseen), assignments, vivas, presentations, practical demonstrations, projects, teaching sessions, report forms and the viewing by others of any 'performance'.

These assessments will range from the informal to the formal, including interviews for change of position, individual performance reviews or as part of preceptorship or clinical supervision situations. Appraisals are both self-assessment and assessment of performance by another while in post, and may occur yearly or in accordance with local policy.

Purdy (1997) states though that 'self-assessment is an important skill to develop since many practitioners may rarely have their professional performance appraised overtly once they have finished their basic professional education'.

Whichever form or means of assessment is used, Brown (1997) states that assessment for learning should:

- accommodate individual differences between students
- clearly explain the purpose of the assessment to all
- provide students with meaningful and useful feedback
- enable students to reflect on their performance
- be an integral part of curriculum design
- involve criteria that are clear, explicit and public
- be of an appropriate amount to be manageable for staff and students
- be demonstrably valid, reliable and consistent.

The wide range of assessment opportunities means that a large number of people can be involved. The following chapter will address this issue.

Conclusion

By the end of this section the reader should be able to:

- list five reasons for having assessment within an educational programme
- discuss the possible links between motivation and assessment
- justify responses to the following situations:

  * Jessica asks for the rationale behind the standard set for her to achieve.

  * Danny asks you why you have to watch and question him on his actions and why you always seem to make negative comments. He illustrates this by saying, 'You said yesterday that I was doing it right but today you tell me to think about observing the patients' facial response when I am talking to them. You did not say that yesterday.'

References and suggested further reading

Brown S (1997) *Innovations in Assessment*. A key note lecture for the Welsh National Board, Cardiff

Brown S, Race P, Smith B (1996) *500 Tips on Assessment*. Kogan Page, London

Child D (1986) *Psychology and the teacher,* 4th edn. Cassell Education, London

College of Occupational Therapists (1989–1991) cited in: Wright CC, Whittington D (1992) *Quality Assurance: An introduction for health care professionals.* Churchill Livingstone, Edinburgh: 8

Cotton J (1995) *The Theory of Assessment. An Introduction.* Kogan Page, London

Girot EA (1993) Assessment of competence in clinical practice — a review of the literature. *Nurse Ed Today* **13**: 83–90

Honey P, Mumford A (1986) *Manual of Learning Styles.* Honey and Mumford, Berkshire

Klug B (1974) *Pro Profiles.* NUS Publications, London

Knowles MS (1984) *The Adult Learner: A Neglected Species,* 2nd edn. Gulf Publishing Co, Houston

Lorentzon M, ed (1992) *Professionalism and Professionalisation.* Distance Learning Centre, South Bank University, London

Maslow A (1971) *The Farther Reaches of Human Nature.* Penguin, Harmondsworth

McClelland DC, Atkinson JW, Clark RA *et al* (1953) The achievement Motive. Appleton Century Crofts, New York. Cited in: Hilgard ER, Atkinson RL, Atkinson RC (1979) *Introduction to Psychology,* 7th edn. Harcourt Brace Jovanovich, New York

Purdy M (1997) The problem of self-assessment in nurse education. *Nurse Ed Today* **17**: 135–139

Quinn FM (1995) *Principles and Practice of Nurse Education,* 3rd edn. Chapman Hall, London

Rowntree D (1987) *Assessing Students: How shall we know them?* Kogan Page, London

Weiner B (1979) A theory of motivation for some classroom experiences. *J Educ Psychol* **71**: 3–25

3
Who can assess?

This chapter will look at **who** can assess in nursing by examining the following roles:

- mentor
- assessor
- preceptor
- clinical supervisor

It may be helpful to read some of the articles referred to in the reading list (marked with an asterisk*) at the end of this chapter before commencing this next activity.

Activity 15

Complete the following and try and identify the similarities and differences between these terms:

	Mentor	**Preceptor**	**Assessor**	**Clinical supervisor**
role				
function				
responsibilities				
qualifications				
qualities				

You may find that you have more than one definition for a term; look critically at the different interpretations.

There are several definitions of the terms mentor, preceptor, assessor and clinical supervisor and not all are consistent with the way that they are incorporated into practice.

Looking at them in more detail it can also be seen that there are overlaps and confusion between the terms. The following section consists of an analytical discussion of the terms and ends with the authors' suggestions, although it is recognised that these conclusions are not definitive.

Mentor

The term appears to be derived from the name of the friend whom Odysseus put in charge of his household when he left for Troy. The friend, Mentor, was the advisor for young Telemachus, Odysseus' son.

Definitions of the term mentor include:

An experienced professional nurturing and guiding the novitiate.

(Butterworth, 1992)

A relationship lasting several years, encompassing choice, emotional ties and sponsorship.

(Donovan, 1990)

Three roles: the inspirer, the investor, the supporter.

(Darling, 1984)

An appropriately qualified and experienced first level nurse/midwife/or health visitor who, by example and facilitation, guides, assists and supports the student in learning new skills, adopting new behaviour and acquiring new attitudes.

(ENB, 1993)

An individual who has an understanding of the context of the student's learning experience and is selected by the student for the purpose of providing guidance and support.

(ENB, 1994)

A mentor is willing to invest time and energy over many years.

(Peutz, 1985)

The conclusions that may be drawn from these definitions are that a mentor may be chosen for you, or by you, that they are generally older and wiser and are turned to for help of all descriptions over varying periods of time.

Anyone can have a mentor although the English National Board (ENB) tends to indicate that mentors are only for the pre-registration students.

However, questions can be asked as to whether a mentor can be an assessor, and also how a mentor differs from a preceptor.

Preceptor

The United Kingdom Central Council (UKCC) (1993) defines a preceptor as:

An experienced first level nurse/midwife/health visitor who acts as a supporter and colleague for a newly registered practitioner or a practitioner re-entering nursing practice. The period of preceptorship should average four months.

The UKCC further states that by 1993 all areas should have introduced preceptorship as a matter of good practice.

The role of the preceptor is seen to encompass:

- orientation to the work environment
- teaching, particularly with regard to the routine work of the clinical area
- support and guidance through new experiences.

Questions still remain as to whether a mentor or preceptor can be an assessor.

* Can either give advice without doing some form of assessment?
* Will the assessment be compromised because of the special relationship between mentor/preceptor and student?

Assessor

This is a formal role with responsibility for judging the level of attainment of a pre- or post-registration student. For continuous assessment of practice the assessor must be based in a clinical area.The ENB (1994) states that an assessor is:

An appropriately qualified and experienced first level nurse/ midwife/health visitor who has undertaken preparation to develop skills in facilitating student learning, supervising practice and assessing the student's level of attainment related to the stated outcomes of the programme.

The assessor should also have some form of recognised instruction prior to completing assessment of others.

This instruction may take the form of recognised study days or the ENB 997/998 course on teaching and assessing in clinical practice.

When exactly a nurse undertakes a course or becomes an assessor may require some clarification, especially with regard to the term 'experienced'. Often, newly qualified staff are asked to complete placement assessment forms. Somers-Smith and Race (1997) state the involvement of recently qualified midwives as assessors risks compromising reliability on three counts:

- their clinical competence has yet to be challenged in a variety of situations
- their academic standards may vary from the current course
- restriction in course length for preparation as an assessor has led to insufficient depth and breadth of skills of teaching and assessing.

This situation would appear to need clarification to prevent the problem of inexperienced staff assessing and making judgements on others.

Also needing clarification is the fact that in clinical practice there appears to be a need for three members of staff, all of whom are first level nurses, one a mentor, one a preceptor, and one an assessor.

Staffing levels on the ward may preclude these roles being invested in separate individuals and often staff are functioning as all three in one. Chandler (1991) identifies a potential problem here in that 'a system that relies on the goodwill and availability of adequately prepared practitioners risks unacceptable compromises in standards of practice'.

Activity 16

Check your list of the qualities required for each role and consider whether one person could fulfil all these roles?

If one person could fulfil all roles this could give rise to a system which is more representative of clinical supervision.

Clinical supervision

Clinical supervision is described as:

A formal process of professional support and learning which enables individual practitioners to develop knowledge and competence, assume responsibility for their own practice and enhance consumer protection and safety of care in complex clinical situations.

(Department of Health, 1993)

An exchange between practising professionals to enable the development of professional skills.

(Butterworth & Faugier, 1992)

The Department of Health document (1993) outlines five implicit themes relevant to the development of the concept of clinical supervision:

* Recognition of developments within the nursing profession, for example, the move from task orientation to total patient care.
* Nurses' individual accountability. 'Personal and professional accountability of individual nurses has become an established practice within the profession since the introduction of the first Code of Professional Conduct in 1983.'
* Nursing developing as a profession. Supervision will assist the process of socialising staff into the values and beliefs, as well as clinical knowledge, of the profession.
* Recent developments such as those found in research and theoretical underpinnings of nursing practice.
* Recognition of other professions — acknowledgement that other professions have a formal structure of clinical supervision.

Defining clinical supervision does not give a clear idea of its application to practice. There appears to be a need for supervision as stated by the Department of Health. Aggleton *et al* (1987) further state that 'there is an explicit assumption that it will assist in the application of nursing theory to practice'. However, Faugier and Butterworth (1993) conclude that, 'clinical supervision has had little impact on the reality of nursing practice or education'.

Examining the term **supervisor** more closely reveals interpretations of a manager or an administrator, possibly not a nurse. Other interpretations may lead to a supervisor being someone who directly views another's performance ensuring that it is to the correct standard. This could mean that the supervisor needs to be a qualified nurse. In other words, a skilled person helping a person less skilled in a particular activity to achieve competence. This would tend to give an indication that the supervisor is more senior rather than a peer.

Supervision can be seen to have four main functions:

- education
- support
- management
- development of self-awareness

The role of a supervisor according to Morris *et al* (1988) includes:

- role model
- supervisor
- facilitator
- assessor

The role of the supervisor is to ensure that relevant experience is provided so that the students can achieve their learning outcomes.

According to Jowett *et al* (1992) supervisors perceive their role as teaching and observing the students' progress, supervising their work, guiding the student towards educational opportunities, being a resource for information, advice and counselling.

Andrusyn and Maltby (1993) state that students see a supervisor as someone:

- *who can be used as a sounding board*
- *who will steer them in the right direction*
- *with whom they can discuss areas of specific interest*
- *with whom they can have a non-prescriptive relationship which is creative and which encourages responsibility.*

Students particularly value the following aspects of clinical supervision (Fowler, 1996):

- *the ethos of a positive learning environment*
- *the non-prescriptive supervisor who can transfer her skills without belittling the learner.*

Three terms are commonly used to encompass the concept of supervision: mentor, preceptor, clinical supervisor.

The supervisor/supervisee relationship often becomes one of professional respect and mutual recognition of knowledge and expertise, even though clinical supervision may be completed by peers.

The following diagram illustrates a summary of expectations of the function, role and value of the clinical supervisor according to the Department of Health (1993), Morris *et al* (1988) and Fowler (1996).

DoH, 1993	Morris *et al*, 1988	Fowler, 1996
Function	**Role**	**Valued as**
education	role model	expert working in clinical area
management	facilitator	non-prescriptive supervisor who transfers skills
support	supervisor	does not belittle learner
development of self-awareness	assessor	

The ENB sees the roles of supervisor and assessor as being combined to aid the concept of continuous assessment.

So why is the use of clinical supervision limited and confined to specific disciplines? Is not a mentor, preceptor or assessor doing clinical supervision?

Activity 17

Refer to *A Vision for the Future* document (DoH, 1993) definition, found on pages 24 and 25 and think about the possibility/problems of clinical supervision in your clinical area.

Now compare your thoughts with the work of Jowett *et al* (1992), who list the following as some of the difficulties with supervision:
- supervising more than one individual at a time
- differing styles of paperwork
- increasing managerial responsibilities
- conflict between performing work at speed and teaching student at his/her pace.

Another difficulty could be having the time to do clinical supervision properly.

In looking at these difficulties related to clinical supervision there are possibly many similarities to problems related to mentorship, preceptorship and assessment.

The following is a possible means of managing supervision.

Supervision starts with an introduction between the student and his/her 'supervisor'. The introduction should include a discussion which centres on the student, remembering that the student:
- is an adult who has some previous learning experiences
- comes with some expectations
- needs some guidance as to what to expect to learn.

This discussion should give rise to the development of an individual learning programme or **learning contract**.

This will require the supervisor to know about the previous experience of the supervisee (qualified nurse, student nurse or care assistant) and the anticipated/required/expected experience.

Learning contracts

Learning contracts are not legal documents but are a useful way for learning outcomes to be stated and discussed to assist in their achievement. The contract is an individually designed learning plan which is negotiated between an assessor and assessee.

The contract needs to set achievable, realistic and measurable targets within an agreed timescale.

With targets set it must be remembered to ensure that they are achieved, so meeting times need to be negotiated to check on progress made to date.

It is important to incorporate aspects that will help motivation, such as realistic achievement with appropriate acknowledgement.

Learning contracts can be used in a variety of clinical practice contexts, for example, with:

1) The preceptor: discussing the nurse's learning needs on newly qualifying or starting in a new clinical environment.

2) The mentor/ assessor: with the student needing specific guidance to achieve a learning outcome of a continuous practical assessment or competencies document.

3) Individually: as a student takes responsibility for his/her own lifelong learning as strengths and weaknesses are personally identified.

4) Individually: for the development of a personal profile for PREP or accreditation of prior achievement purposes.

A learning contract is also useful if a student is having difficulty in achieving continuous practical assessment objectives/competencies. The learning outcomes would be listed accordingly.

In whichever context the contract is drawn up, the following issues should be addressed:

- objectives or learning outcomes to be achieved
- where specific responsibilities lie
- which activities are required to achieve the objectives or outcomes
- how outcomes will be evaluated
- what the rewards will be.

When setting up a learning contract it is important to identify, in order of priority, the individual's self-learning needs and the action needed to meet them. These learning needs may have been clarified with a supervisor.

Example of a learning contract

This example uses a common situation of a newly qualified nurse starting in a new clinical area, possibly in a new trust.

Learning outcomes	Learning resources/ strategies to be used	Evidence	Date for achievement	Signatures and date of achievement
To be orientated to the hospital	Visits organised	Be able to visit key departments, eg. theatre, pharmacy, blood bank, without direction	By end of second week	
To be able to name different members of the ward team	Ward reports, ward rounds, Jane's leaving party	Preceptor will ask questions and clarify knowledge	By end of second week, ie. 16 January	
To be familiar with the trust's drug adminis-tration policies and the specific drugs used on the ward	Trust Policy Documents, UKCC (1992) Standards for the Adminis-tration of Medicines. Act as 2nd administrator of drugs. Act as 1st administrator of drugs	Give brief explanation of drugs to preceptor/patient as appropriate	End of 3rd week Beginning of 4th week Beginning of 6th week	

When setting a learning contract there are likely to be many other areas of identified weakness which will need attention. The important thing is the priority order so that safety can be maintained.

There are certain requirements without which a contract becomes quite meaningless.

- the student or assessee should be self-motivated and self- directed
- the outcomes/objectives should be clearly identified
- the means by which these outcomes will be evaluated/assessed should be stated
- the time scale should be stated and be realistic and achievable
- the contract should be written, signed and dated.

The learning contract documents can be written in a variety of formats with detail to suit the situation.

The folowing example uses a student on a clinical placement in his/her pre-registration period.

Outcome	Resources	Evidence	Date of completion
Provide a patient with relevant health education	Clinical area Nursing staff	Discuss two observed situations of patients receiving health education	Week 1
	Clinical area Patient's notes	Identify a patient requiring health education	End of week 1
	Ward resources Library Health education department	Review and collate suitable health education literature	2nd week
		Present the information to mentor	3rd week
		Present information to the patient	4th week

Once completed the contract needs to be kept in the preceptee's/ assessee's portfolio. This evidence, substantiated by the preceptor's signature, can then be used for accreditation purposes.

Conclusion

At the end of this section the reader should be able to:
- define and critically analyse the terms mentor, preceptor, assessor and clinical supervisor
- compare responses to activity 15 (*page 21*) with the following:

	Mentor	Preceptor	Assessor	Clinical supervisor
role	support	guidance	observer	advice/ guidance
function	supervise	example	judge	oversee
responsibilities	guide/ protect	enable	ensure safety	develop staff

qualifications	1 day (min) course	2 day (min) course	recognised course, eg. 997/998	management clinical/ assessing
qualities	approach-able	competent	objective	responsive

- identify four possible problems linked to each term listed in the above box as it is applied to your own clinical area
- discuss the rationale for responses to the following situations:

  * Jessica has read widely about mentorship and clinical supervision and she asks you to explain which system you are using in your clinical area and why. She has an assignment to write on this subject.

  * Danny has complained because his mentor, who he dislikes, has now completed his assessment form and not given him a very good result. He asks you why his mentor should be assessing him. **Alternatively:**

  * Danny's mentor has gone on holiday and left you with a note asking you to give Danny his report. You have not been involved in his supervision but have heard about his reputation for being casual.

References and suggested further reading

Aggleton P, Allen M, Montgomery S (1987) Developing a system for the continuous assessment of practical nursing skills. *Nurse Ed Today* 7: 158–164

Andrusyn M, Maltby H (1993) Building on strengths through preceptorship. *Nurse Ed Today* 13: 277–281

*Armitage P, Burnard P (1991) Mentors or preceptors? Narrowing the theory–practice gap. *Nurse Ed Today* 11: 225–229

*Bains L (1996) Preceptorship: A review of the literature. *J Adv Nurs* 24: 104–107

Barlow S (1991) Impossible Dream. *Nurs Times* 87(1): 53–54

Butterworth T (1992) Clinical supervision as an emerging idea in nursing. Cited in: Butterworth T, Faugier J (1992) *Clinical Supervision and Mentorship in Nursing*. Chapman and Hall, London: 3–17

*Butterworth T, Bishop V, Carson J (1996) First steps towards evaluating clinical supervision in nursing and health visiting. I. Theory, policy and practice development. A review. *J Clin Nurs* 5: 127–132

Carlisle C (1991) The Value of Contract Learning. *Nurs* 4 (26): 22–24

Chandler (1991) Reforming nurse education 2 — Implications for teachers and students. *Nurse Ed Today* **11**: 89–93

Child D (1986) *Psychology and the Teacher*, 4th edn. Cassell Education, London

Cotton J (1995) *The Theory of Assessment. An Introduction.* Kogan Page, London

Darling L (1984) What do nurses want in a mentor? *J Nurs Admin* **14**(10): 42–44

Department of Health (1989) *Caring for People — Community Care in the Next Decade and Beyond.* HMSO, London

Department of Health (1992) *The Health of the Nation: A Strategy for Health in England.* HMSO, London

Department of Health (1993) *A Vision for the Future. The Nursing Midwifery and Health Visiting Contribution to Health and Health Care.* HMSO, London

Department of Health (1995) *The Patient's Charter and You.* HMSO, London

Donovan J (1990) The concept and role of mentor. *Nurse Ed Today* **10**: 294–298

English National Board (1993) *Regulations and Guidelines for the Approval of Institutions and Courses.* English National Board for Nursing, Midwifery and Health Visiting, London

English National Board (1994) Changes to Regulations and Guidelines for the Approval of Institutions and Courses. *ENB News* **14**

Ersser S (1991) A search for the therapeutic dimension of nurse–patient interaction. Cited in: McMahon R, Pearson A (eds) (1991) *Nursing as Therapy.* Chapman Hall, London: 43–84

Faugier J, Butterworth T (1993) *Clinical Supervision — A Position Paper.* School of Nursing Studies, University of Manchester, Manchester

*Fowler J (1996) How to use models of clinical supervision in practice. *Nurs Standard* **10**(29): 42–47

*Fowler J (1996) The organisation of clinical supervision within the nursing profession: a review of the literature. *J Adv Nurs* **23**: 471–478

Grant P (1993) Contract Learning. *Nurs Times* **84**(46): 25–27

Jowett S, Walton I, Payne S (1992) *Implementing Project 2000 — An Interim Report.* National Foundation for Educational Research in England and Wales, Windsor

*Maggs C (1994) Mentorship in nursing and midwifery education: Issues for research. *Nurse Ed Today* **14**: 22–29

Maslin-Prothereo S (ed) (1997) *Baillière's Study Skills for Nurses.* Baillière Tindall, RCN, London: Appendix B

Morris N, John G, Keen T (1988) Mentors: learning the ropes. *Nurs Times* **84**(46): 24–27

Peutz B (1985) Learning the ropes from a mentor. *Nurs Success Today* **2** (6): 11–13

Quinn FM (1995) *Principles and Practice of Nurse Education,* 3rd edn. Chapman Hall, London

Somers-Smith MJ, Race A (1997) Assessment of clinical skills in midwifery: some ethical and practical problems. *Nurse Ed Today* **17**(6): 449–453

Sutcliffe L (1993) Leaps of Knowledge. *Nurs Times* **89**(42): 34–36

United Kingdom Central Council (1993) *The Council's Position Concerning a Period of Support and Preceptorship* . Registrar's Letter 1/1993. Annexe one. United Kingdom Central Council for Nursing, Midwifery and Health Visiting, London

United Kingdom Central Council for Nursing, Midwifery and Health Visiting (1992) *Standards for the Administration of Medicines.* UKCC, London

4

The 'when' of assessment

Course assessment of theory and practice occurs at various times. As previously discussed, individuals assess each other all the time. This is implicit in this chapter which will discuss aspects of 'when' formal assessment occurs and will address the terms formative and summative as related to assessment.

Activity 18

Identify when you have been assessed on a nursing course and the types of assessment undertaken.

Timing of assessments varies tremendously in courses. The kinds of assessment included could be:

Theory	Practice
Essays	Ward reports
Objective tests	Ward based assessments
Assignments	Individual assessment
Verbal tests	Competency achievement
Modular tests	Continuous assessment
Examinations	

On page 1 the definition of assessment by Rowntree (1987) suggested that interaction in assessment is either 'direct or indirect'. Direct assessment has been discussed as assessment that is seen and heard or observed at the actual time of assessment. In other words, it is important that direct assessment is recognised as such, as these assessments require an assessor to be present.

Indirect assessment may be seen as the assessment that occurs without the need for a meeting of the student and the assessor.

Activity 19

Can you identify which of the above types of assessment are direct assessments and which are indirect?

Direct assessments can generally include all assessments of practice. They also include verbal tests such as *viva voces*.

Indirect assessments are assessments where the student and the assessor do not have to meet or, in fact, have any contact except for the submission of the work to be assessed. These assessments could include a written assignment or examination paper.

Apart from assessment being an interaction that can be either 'direct' or 'indirect' there are other terms that can be used in the classification of assessment. These include the terms 'formative', 'summative' and 'continuous' assessment.

Formative assessment

This is directed towards developing the student and contributing to his/her growth and is:

a continuing and systematic review of a student to determine the degree of mastery of a given learning task and to help the student and teacher to focus on particular learning necessary to achieve mastery.

(Kenworthy and Nicklin, 1989)

Bradshaw (1989) states:

a formative process is one of recording, reporting and commenting upon a student's work, personal qualities and social skills as s/he progresses. Students can be helped to identify strengths and weaknesses and to develop competence with the principal aim of improving future attainment and development.

Formative assessment should come before summative assessment to allow the student to recognise his/her strengths and weaknesses. However, there may be instances when formative assessment is offered in an educational programme but the student is given the option of whether to accept help and guidance or not.

An example of formative assessment that is offered on many courses is individual tutorials, however the student is given the option of whether they wish to attend.

Formative assessment needs to function to reinforce a student's learning giving the student the opportunity to increase his/her confidence and understanding before a final judgement is made. To enable this to happen, periods of formative assessment need to be planned by the student and the assessor (see the section on *learning contracts and the link to assessment, pages 40–41).*

Summative assessment

This can be described as any attempt to reach an overall description or judgement of a student. Any or all of the previously listed assessment types could be used as the format for summative assessment.

Summative assessment can be described as a generalised assessment of a student's achievement of the objectives for the course as a whole, or for a substantial part of the course. The result of the summative assessment contributes to the grading of the student and their qualification or certificate. Summative assessment must be passed to progress on any given course or to successfully achieve the course outcome.

Activity 20

> Identify the formative and summative components of the last or present course you have attended and consider the benefits or otherwise of both types of assessment.

Many courses whether terminally assessed or continuously assessed have formative and summative elements.

A list of formative and summative assessment within a course could include:

Formative	Summative
presentation	project
literature review	research proposal
tutorials/group discussion	assignment
supervised practice	competencies
mock test questions	examinations

Formative assessment is not always compulsory as in the case of tutorials when the student can select whether s/he would like some help. In the case of practical assessment the student should receive formative assessment before summative assessment to enable him/her to identify weaknesses and take corrective action. The formative and summative assessment of practice may not take place in the same clinical area but may be ongoing from one placement to another.

It is also important to consider whether Bloom's (1956) three components of learning: knowledge, skills and attitudes are being assessed.

Assessment is an integral part of a nursing programme but what should be assessed in order for a nurse to qualify with the UKCC? What information needs to be obtained and interpreted?

This issue is looked at in *chapter 5*, 'How to assess'.

A further consideration is the fact that nurses do not assess just other nurses: they may also be involved in the assessment of other staff including healthcare assistants.

This next section will look briefly at assessment of National Vocational Qualifications (NVQs).

Assessment of National Vocational Qualifications (NVQs)

NVQs are acquired by achieving competent performance which is assessed to a nationally agreed standard. These standards reflect the expected performance of the person in the workplace and as such are written as outcomes.

For this section, the person involved in taking an NVQ, although recognised as a healthcare worker, will be referred to as an assistant.

There are five levels of achievement that have been identified within the National Vocational Qualifications.

Level 1 concerns the performance of repetitive actions. This performance does not occur within healthcare as, although functions are performed, there are individual variations which can concern venue, equipment or sequence of performance.

Level 2 concerns performance that can be learnt by 'doing' but requires supervision.

Level 3 involves actions that can be performed independently following certain agreed guidelines. NVQ level 3 qualifications can be used as evidence to access nurse training.

Level 4 concerns management issues. This level may be completed by a nurse following registration or by a person not from a nursing background.

Level 5 involves complex competencies across a broad range of unpredictable contexts.

For the healthcare worker/assistant, as with other workers, the NVQ route provides choice.

The choice relates to those aspects that are applicable to the assistant's specific work area at the time.

All NVQs consist of a similar format:
- units of competence
- elements of competence
- performance criteria
- range statements
- knowledge specifications
- evidence requirements.

An assistant commencing an NVQ will be given the relevant documentation and will then agree with the mentor/assessor in the work area the applicability of the units and the appropriate sequence of the units for the individual's need. Considerations for the assistant will relate to the specific area of care, eg. developmental, direct, domicilliary.

Within healthcare the competencies consist of core components and endorsements.

Core components must be completed for each NVQ.

Endorsement units are selected for their relevance to the work area. Each endorsement unit must be taken as appropriate and linked to the core components.

One core component is seen as the value base unit — Unit O — this must be completed with each unit. Unit O is seen as the essential, integral part of each related unit. As a result of the integration of the core components into each unit, the endorsement units are often completed first and then the core components at the end. In this way, much of the work of the core component has been completed during the unit.

If the assistant changes work area, then the appropriate endorsement units with the core components will need to be completed. The assistant may be exempt from an endorsement unit in the new NVQ if s/he has already taken the unit linked to the other area of work. However, core components still require completion as they are linked to the new endorsement unit.

While completing the NVQ the assistant will keep an evidence log of experience and complete a portfolio.

The assistant will receive some theoretical input and consequent study time and may be expected to present aspects of work linked to the unit to others during the study time.

Apart from benefits to the organisation, NVQs should benefit the assistant.

Simosko and Cook (1996) state that NVQs benefit the individual employee and the *'benefits include:*

improved performance

recognition of existing competence

higher self-esteem and self-awareness of skills

increased confidence to participate and "add value" at work

enhanced progression and transfer opportunities

improved management and organisational skills

greater motivation towards personal development.'

Assessment decisions are based on a combination of evidence.

Achievement of performance is assessed as formative assessment rather than summmative, although the assistant is required to reach the competent stage within an agreed set time period. The assessor will work with the assistant, taking the role of mentor plus assessor and advise the assistant on his/her level of performance.

When a competent performance is achieved it is noted and documented.

Assessors of NVQs must:

- be competent in their own area
- have completed a recognised course (eg. TDLB, D32/33)
- have been accepted as an assessor.

Quality and reliability of assessment is monitored by:

1. Internal verification

Internal verifiers monitor the reliability and validity of assessments. An internal verifier will sample the assessor's function during an assessment and in the discussion and completion of documented evidence. They are required to provide a report of the internal NVQ process.

All internal verifiers are required to hold a TDLB unit D34, National Council for Vocational Qualifications (1993).

II. External verification

External verification will be completed by an external verifier who has been appointed to the assessment centre by the awarding body.

External assessors monitor both the centre's equal opportunities practice and assessment process, and also ensure that adequate information systems are available. External verifiers are also responsible for the moderation of portfolios and the assessment process.

McMahon (1994)

Learning contracts and the link to assessment

Learning contracts have been discussed in *chapter 3*. The contract has been shown to be an agreed action between a student and a mentor/ preceptor/clinical supervisor or an assessor. The contract is drawn up with the intended outcome to be achieved. Often a learning contract can be linked to an assessment situation. The student wants to achieve a successful outcome. The example on *page 41* illustrates how formative and summative assessments might be used to achieve a specific learning outcome, such as to be familiar with the trust's drug administration policies and the specific drugs used on the ward.

* At the end of a six-week placement the student wishes to act competently as a first administrator of drugs, under supervision.

* By week five the student intends to be able to give the mentor a brief explanation about the drugs administered to the patients, as appropriate.

A learning contract can be devised around the outcome in more detail as the following example indicates.

Assessment stages are indicated as: formative (f) and summative (s).

The evidence column is linked to the theory of Steinaker and Bell (1979) experiential taxonomy (see *chapter 5*).

Conclusion

At the end of this chapter the reader should be able to:

- review the assessment requirements of students in your own clinical area and identify:
  i) direct and indirect assessment
  ii) formative and summative assessment
- consider your response to the following situations:

  * Jessica has seen you working with a healthcare assistant and has noted that the assistant has completed an aseptic technique and there has been discussion concerning the achievement of this outcome. She asks you why she cannot try to achieve NVQ competencies.

  * Danny complains again about his poor report. This time he tells you that no one discussed his performance with him at any time during his six week allocation. He had to ask for the assessment to be completed on his last day. If he had not asked, he did not feel he would have been given the report then.

Learning resources	Evidence	Assessment
Patient prescription sheets	List of commonly used drugs for clinical area	
	Notes on drugs, their actions and their normal dose	End of week 1 (f) Discussion on drugs and their actions
	Exposure to drug administration	
	Review drug administration procedure	End of week 3 (f) Assessment to observe if the level of identification has been achieved
	Participate in drug administration as 1st administrator demonstrating level of identification	End of week 5 (f) observed/supervised assessment of drug administration with questioning on drugs and their actions and regulations
	Participate in drug administration as 1st administrator demonstrating level of internalisation	During week 6 (s) Observed/supervised assessment of drug administration with questioning on drugs and their actions and regulations

References and further reading

Bloom B (1956) *Taxonomy of Educational Objectives: The Classification of Educational Goals. Handbook One: Cognitive Domain.* McKay, New York

Bradshaw PL (1989) *Teaching and Assessing in Clinical Practice.* Prentice Hall, New York

Clifford C (1994) Assessment of Clinical Practice and the Role of the Nurse Teacher. *Nurse Ed Today* **14**: 272–279

Cotton J (1995) *The Theory of Assessment. An Introduction.* Kogan Page, London

Day M (1992) Quality training for HCAs. *Nurs Times* **89**(24): 32–34

Greaves K (1993) Exploring the issues. National Vocational Qualifications. *Br J Theatre Nurs* June 3, 3: 14–19, 22–27

Jarvis P, Gibson S (1997) *The Teacher Practitioner in Nursing, Midwifery, Health Visiting and the Social Services,* 2nd edn. Stanley Thornes, Cornwall

Kenworthy N, Nicklin P (1989) *Teaching and Assessing in Nursing Practice. An experiential approach.* Scutari, London

McMahon C (1994) At the front of the NVQ. *Nurs Management* 1(4): 22–23

NCVQ (1993) Access and equal opportunity. *Care Standards* 2(2): 1–4

NCVQ (1993) The awarding bodies' common accord. NVCQ, London

Quinn FM (1995) *Principles and Practice of Nurse Education,* 3rd edn. Chapman Hall, London

Raper J (1992) NVQs; where are they leading? *Occ Health* 4(12): 369–372

Rowntree D (1987) *Assessing Students: How shall we know them?* Kogan Page, London

Simosko S, Cook C (1996) *Applying APL Principles in Flexible Assessment: a practical guide,* 2nd edn. Kogan Page, London

Steinaker NW, Bell MR (1979) *The Experimental Taxonomy.* Academic Press, New York

Storey L (1995) Nurse education goes better with formula NVQ. *Nurs Management* 1(10): 20–22

5

How to assess

This chapter will look at criteria for assessment and include a discussion on validity, reliability, discrimination and practicability. In addition, assessment tools and the role of the assessor will be examined.

Assessment criteria must ensure validity, reliability, discrimination and practicality. These aspects will be emphasised as important to any type of assessment.

Validity according to Quinn (1995) is 'the extent to which the test measures what it is designed to measure'.

In nursing, any test given must measure whether someone is suitable to be a nurse.

The way this is being made possible for nursing is by the achievement of competencies at increasing levels in order to achieve the responsibilities of a nurse as stated in the Nurses, Midwives and Health Visitors Act 1979/1992/1997.

The test or assessment must be justifiable in terms of the intended outcome. Not only must the assessment be justified and valid but the components of an assessment must also be valid and have their rationale justified. As discussed on *page 10* there must be a valid reason behind the questions asked in assessment. This valid reason for asking the questions must be linked to a reliable decision made from the answers. In other words, not only must the assessor ask the right questions, but also the right method of assessment must be selected to enable the required answer to be given.

Many discussions have occurred between markers of students' scripts, for example, when a student has written that s/he would give the patient 100mg morphine IM, does this indicate a written mistake or an error that would be made in practice? The decision to pass or fail must depend on the rest of the answer which will provide extra evidence of knowledge and understanding.

In reading this example did you think that this might have been a printing error — 10 not 100mg, or did you read it as ten rather than one hundred. It is sometimes easy to make the mistake on paper but, in practice, would a nurse draw up ten ampoules of morphine to give to a patient?

Take, for example, the following situation:

Scenario 8

A student is giving a controlled drug to a patient. As part of the assessment you ask the student what are the three most important indications of an excess of morphine. This could be a valid question as you want to assess that the student would recognise signs of morphine overdose. However, does s/he pass or fail if s/he gives one right answer or all three?

This raises the question as to whether drug doses should be tested in practice with appropriate equipment or on paper in a written examination/assignment/care study. However, it is important that the expected answers should be agreed by assessors in order to try and achieve maximum reliability.

Reliability according to Quinn (1995) is 'the consistency with which a test measures what it is designed to measure'.

In other words, can any assessor using the same tool and set of circumstances come up with the same result and can the same assessor using the same test on another occasion come up with the same result?

An illustration of the kind of problem that can arise in measurement was provided quite by chance by a six year old who, in response to the information that an object was a foot long, asked, 'Is that your foot or mine!' The child's understanding of the unit of measurement was clearly not the same as the informer's.

The same units of measurement must be understood and used by both the assessee and the assessor.

Oppenheim (1984) uses the illustration of a clock to clarify the relationship between validity and reliability. A clock is valid if it measures 'true' time and reliable if it does so consistently. It would be invalid as a tool if it showed the wrong time and unreliable if it was sometimes slow and sometimes fast. This also illustrates the fact that a tool can have poor validity while being reliable, as a clock that is consistently ten minutes fast.

Assessment should in all circumstances measure what it says it is measuring.

Discrimination

Assessment should also discriminate. It should identify the difference between a satisfactory and an unsatisfactory performance.

This can involve a decision concerning whether assessment is measured by criterion, norm or ipsative measurement.

Criterion assessment involves comparing the student's performance with a predetermined set of criteria which is often related to the course expectations and the stage in the course. Many of the assessment tools used in nursing both to assess patients, eg. the Norton score and to assess nurses, eg. the continuous assessment practical report are examples of criterion assessment.

Norm reference assessment involves comparing one student's performance with the level set by other students. This is not commonly used in nurse education but one example may be the interview criteria when a decision has to be made between several interviewees. Six candidates are interviewed but there are only four places, therefore a decision has to be made. In some forms of written examination a selection may be made as to how many students might pass. The pass mark has not been fixed at a certain level. Instead, if 50% of the group obtain marks of 45% and above, the pass mark may be agreed as that. Alternatively if 50% of the group had a mark of 55% the pass mark may be set at 55%. In clinical practice there is a tendency to compare the performance of students at the same stage in training which could be considered as norm assessment, but the assessment form has predetermined criteria making it criterion assessment. If norm reference assessment were to be carried out in clinical practice there would be a serious possibility that poor performance could become an acceptable 'norm'.

Ipsative assessment, according to Cotton (1995), 'measures individual improvement by comparing the grade or level at the start and the finish of a learning programme'. This may be done if the student has the same practical assessment form completed in each clinical area graded on levels of competence. Correct completion of this form should demonstrate improvement, which may be recorded along the lines of the Steinaker and Bell (1979) theory, (see *pages 58–59* for application of this theory). However, in practice there can be problems with this type of assessment as the opportunities are not always available in each area, also students might achieve a high level of attainment in some aspects early on in their training and then have to achieve that same level throughout the rest of their training. Also, it may be extremely discouraging, ie. demotivating, for beginner students to achieve very low grades on early tests.

This raises the question of consistent performance or 'good days and poor days'.

Consider the following with regard to punctuality and attendance. In this incident, the reader needs to consider that the student used in the example is a paid and employed member of staff.

Activity 21

Decide what is acceptable. What is satisfactory or unsatisfactory performance? A student is on a two week (10 day) clinical placement. How often can the student be late/absent?

Is it possible that a student can be late/absent 10% of the time and still pass? Each week the student would work five days on and two days off. Therefore, this would be one day in a 10 day placement.

Would such an apparently high level of absenteeism matter so much on a 40 day placement?

If the pass/fail criteria was just a pass or fail then one day may be a clear decision **but** if the criteria awarded was an A, B, or C to pass then the situation changes.

A = on time   present every day
B = late   absent once
C = late   absent twice

The student would therefore pass with a ratio of two days late/absent in ten days.

Other issues that may need to be considered with lateness or absenteeism are:

* Whether the student is late/absent with a good reason or not. Does the assessor allow more lateness if the reason is sound?

* Is lateness a more serious problem than absenteeism, or the reverse?

Part of the answer to the question regarding absenteeism may be found in a local policy. If the policy states that absenteeism without notification is a disciplinary situation, this may guide the assessor's action. Remember that if there is an absenteeism policy then the student may only be allowed to be absent without notification twice and then s/he may receive a final disciplinary warning and may even be dismissed. This would obviously constitute a failure.

Prior to the assessment process the student should have been told of the expected performance, that is s/he will have been advised about the policy. The first instance of absence should have been discussed with the student and any action to help the student taken. This would constitute the formative stage. If the student was absent for a second time then it can be looked at as summative assessment, providing that the student had received the necessary help and guidance with regard to the first absence. Absenteeism may only be allowed on one occasion to allow for a satisfactory assessment.

However, for assessment to discriminate and therefore be reliable, assessors must agree to the criteria.

Activity 22

> Question your own views and those of others on this particular issue of lateness /absenteeism and examine how discrimination can be achieved to allow for reliability.

Practicality

Assessment needs to be applicable within the confines of the situation. It must be **practical** in time and resources. Assessment of practical situations is often completed on a one to one basis with one assessor observing a student. Some assessments not only require the assessor to be present for extended periods of time, eg. a shift, but also to be present only as an observer/assessor of the student's performance, therefore unable to perform any other activities during the time of observation of one student. During this time of extended observation the student may be required to carry out some activities that bear no relevance to the actual assessment in progress, eg. the student may be asked to assist another member of staff in the care of his/her patient. Also during the assessment period the student might be required to carry out aspects of care that are not directly related to the present assessment. To attain maximum practicality the environment, patient expectations for care and time period of assessment need some degree of control.

Ross *et al* (1988) state that clinical assessment in clinical areas leads to a broad number of variables which alter the assessment situation and the complexity of the assessment from one student to another. Control of the assessment situation may therefore allow for a consistent testing of each student through a wide variety of controlled situations. This may make assessment more manageable/practicable (see *page 85* on the objective structured clinical assessment).

Ross *et al* (1988) support the notion of assessment of students in larger numbers and in a variety of situations.

Two assessment tools will now be looked at and critically discussed with regard to their validity, reliability, discrimination and practicality. The two tools selected are not examples from the assessment of students but the assessment of patients. They have been chosen due to the fact that they illustrate the points. The principles within these forms of assessment can be applied to all the types of assessment of nurses discussed so far.

The **Apgar score** (1953) is a tool to measure the physical state of an infant.

Look at the assessment tool and examine the aspects that the tool indicates to be assessed. Consider whether they are all consistent with a description of a physical state.

(Please note that only a section of the assessment tool is shown.)

Sign	0	1	2
heart rate	absent	slow <100	>100
respiratory effort	absent	weak cry	good strong cry
colour	blue/pale	body pink extremities blue	completely pink

The aspects to assess are described as signs. The signs to be looked for are all physical properties, eg. heart rate, colour. Therefore, the tool could be said to be valid — it is measuring what it should.

Look now at whether the tool is reliable. Would everyone come up with the same results?

For example, what score would you give for a pulse of 100?

If the results are liable to be different, eg. a score of 1 or 2 then the result is not reliable. This may indicate a problem either with the assessment tool or with the assessor using the tool.

The assessment tool may need to be made reliable.

In this case a score of 1 for a pulse of 99 or less; 2 for 100 or more.

Now consider whether this tool will allow a nurse to identify clearly a satisfactory or unsatisfactory physical state. The resulting score should be able to discriminate between a satisfactory or unsatisfactory physical state. For example, a score of 0 would indicate an extremely poor physical state but there can also be interim scores when the decision between poor and good may be a little unclear.

Practicality would consider when to use the Apgar tool and its ease of use. As with most assessment tools the assessor needs to have the skills/ knowledge to use the tool. So, with the Apgar score the assessor will have been taught at some time how to complete an Apgar assessment. This instruction will allow for speed of use.

One reason why an assessment may not be practicable may be related to the time it takes to complete. However the Apgar score must be used quickly and therefore has been designed to allow assessment of the infant's physical state within a minute of birth and five minutes after birth.

Activity 23

Look now at the Norton score below:
1. State what the tool is measuring.
2. Critically analyse whether the tool is reliable and practicable.

Norton scale

A Physical condition		B Mental condition		C Activity		D Mobility		E Continence	
good	4	alert	4	ambulant	4	full	4	not	4
fair	3	apathetic	3	walk/help	3	slightly limited	3	occasion-ally	3
poor	2	confused	2	chairbound	2	very limited	2	usually/ urine	2
very bad	1	stuporous	1	bedfast	1	immobile	1	doubly	1

The validity of the Norton score is open to question. When using the tool on a patient a resultant score will be achieved but does this score purely indicate that this patient is at risk of developing pressure sores? The score can indicate that the patient has experienced a series of changes in activity and mental state. The tool does not discriminate between a variety of situations. Part of the reason for not discriminating purely to indicate patients at risk of pressure sores is that some vital indicators are not included in the tool. These indicators could be the patient's dietary state or general medical condition or the medication that he is taking. These are all aspects that could have a bearing on a patient's risk of developing pressure sores.

The Norton score is said to be easy to understand and quick to use, making it practicable, but does this make it reliable? Reliability is linked with discrimination and questions the criteria to be assessed. The difference between a fair, poor and very bad physical state or one which is slightly limited or very limited may be difficult to determine. Differences in interpretation of these categories can lead to an unreliable assessment tool.

If the validity and reliability of the Norton score are in question, its ability to discriminate will also be in question. That is, the Norton score will give a quantitative result but does this clearly indicate the person's risk of developing a pressure sore? The Norton score is not widely used in practice now. It has been used here only as an example.

The pressure sore risk indicator used more widely in practice is the Waterlow score. The validity and reliability of this assessment tool may also be questioned but, due to the wider range of applicable factors assessed, it is able to give a more discriminatory result.

Activity 24

Look at two forms of assessment which are used in your clinical areas. Critically examine whether these tools are valid and/or reliable.

The next section examines the assessment of a nurse. This involves determining what is a valid nursing assessment.

It may be possible to begin to define an assessment situation and tool by examining the overall intent of nurse education.

The primary aim of nurse education is to provide education to maintain and develop a **competent** practitioner.

A competent practitioner or competence of practice requires further definition:

Competence is the possession and development of sufficient skills, knowledge, appropriate attitudes and experience for successful performance in life roles.

(Further Education Curriculum Unit, 1984)

Beaumont (1996) states that competence is,

... the ability to apply knowledge, understanding and skills in performing to the standards required in employment, including solving problems and meeting changing demands.

Within nursing there are a tremendous number of skills to be performed. These skills can range from psychomotor skills to numeracy skills, to communication skills and include the skills of assessment and problem solving and the skills of management.

How many of these skills is a nurse expected to be competent at and how are they to be assessed?

Knowledge acquisition is essential, however the range and depth of knowledge requires some clarification.

The Nurses, Midwives and Health Visitors Act 1979/1992/1997 gives an overall indication of the outcome of nurse education, but again, how much, how specifically and to what depth can a nurse be assessed?

'Appropriate attitude' raises the question as to what is an appropriate or professional attitude and how an attitude can be assessed. If an attitude is assessed according to the assessor's personal expectations this will lead to unreliability and extreme subjectivity. If the attitude of one nurse is compared to the attitude of another nurse then this could be norm referencing. However, these means of assessing an attitude do not necessarily give an accurate result. An agreed set of expectations or criteria (criterion referencing) may give a clearer, more reliable assessment.

However, according to Benner (1984) nursing skills develop in stages. There are five stages:

Novice
    Advanced beginner
        Competent
            Proficient
                Expert

Benner (1984) states that the **competent stage** 'is characterised by conscious, deliberate planning based upon analysis and careful deliberation of situations,' and that, 'the competent nurse is able to identify priorities and manage her work'.

The assessment of nursing practice during pre-registration education needs to meet the criteria of competence, not expert. A registrant may be competent to practise but what are the guidelines for practice? Wright and Whittington (1992) state that competence is the 'presence of necessary knowledge, skills and personal attitudes to allow for the performance of professional tasks'. Professional identification of nursing may be found in the *Code of Professional Conduct.*

The *Code of Professional Conduct* (UKCC, 1992) outlines the responsibilities of the nurse and forms the guidance for assessment.

Other considerations include that nurse assessment must:

- protect the patient
- help the student develop
- identify problem areas for the student
- legitimise the profession.

It must be remembered that nurse assessment cannot pass every student but it must identify those whose practice could jeopardise others, both patients and colleagues.

According to Purdy (1997) nurse education should facilitate:

- individual personal development
- professional selection.

The question of what information needs to be obtained and interpreted still remains.

By law, nurses must successfully achieve the competencies of Rule 18/18A (Nurses, Midwives and Health Visitors Act 1979, 1992 and 1997) in order to register (see *Appendix*).

The *Code of Professional Conduct* (1992) gives guidance as to how to keep within the law, an ethical framework and professional expectations.

Within any course, achievement of knowledge, skills and attitudes can be measured by forms of theoretical and/or practical assessment (see *chapter 4* for discussion on course assessment).

Nursing is multifaceted and, as such, every aspect of a nurse's role in care cannot be assessed or measured in each student undergoing a nursing course. If this was attempted it would lead to a problem of overassessment, to name but one. Therefore, a decision is made on the assessment that the student is required to undertake.

It is implied that assessment consists of some form of measurement. Measurement can result in the awarding of marks which will create a quantitative result; however in the assessment of nursing skills the result is not solely how many patients the nurse has spoken to, but rather the quality of that communication. Many nursing actions require quality and, therefore, for the assessment of practice, qualitative methods of assessment are needed.

Activity 25

Identify one method of measuring the performance of a student nurse. Decide whether the method is assessing quantity or quality or a mixture of both.

In measuring performance the definition of Rowntree (1987) states that assessment includes knowledge, attitudes and skills. These aspects all need to be measured.

Assessing quality or effectiveness is essential but more difficult to determine objectively than quantity assessment. Quality assessment brings into question personal aspects and the problem of subjectivity rather than quantity assessment. The next section looks at assessment related to quality and quantity.

Qualitative and quantitative assessment

Some assessment tools in nursing can be clearly seen to be either quantitative or qualitative, whereas other assessment tools are a mixture.

Quality assessment is measurement against standards/expectations. It involves effectiveness, efficiency and acceptability (Wright and Whittington, 1992).

Quantitative assessment can be found in the numbers of patients seen in a clinic in a day, the number of patient histories that have been taken during a morning shift. Dependence studies are a quantity assessment of the type of care and the amount of nursing time that a patient will require. Staff numbers in relation to patients can also be considered as quantitative assessment.

Policies, procedures and standards can lead to the development of quantity measures, for example, the turning of patients on a two hourly basis. However policies, procedures and standards can indicate the performance required at certain levels and in standard ways and can lead on to qualitative measures. For example, how well the procedure was carried out. Other measures that can be considered involve how the nurse felt about the procedure and, more importantly, how the patient felt. This may include looking at attitudes and in-depth knowledge of rationale, aspects which are not overt. These are issues more related to the qualitative aspects. What a professional attitude may entail, what is being looked for and how it might be measured are issues that are more difficult to answer than how many times, or how many, patients are cared for during a shift.

Attitudes and feelings are often hidden or revealed only to confidants so they cannot be assessed on the basis of actual physical performance. The effectiveness of communication is often the subjective outcome of the assessor's and the assessee's attitudes, feelings and opinions. The effectiveness of patient care can often be measured only by the patient's subjective opinion in the context of many other variables.

Butterworth (1996) discusses that assessment is in the process of change from 'hard' strategies to 'soft'.

'Hard' strategies are assessments such as essays and terminal examinations, but possibly could include the pre-arranged ward based assessments. These forms of assessment were traditionally norm-referenced and could be quantitatively monitored.

'Soft' strategies include continuous assessment, profiles, peer assessment and oral presentations. These forms of assessment are often criterion referenced. The criteria need to relate closely to the specific course. The criteria can relate to a wide range including knowledge, psychomotor and affective skills, thereby assessing qualitative issues. However, they are only as good as the shared standard set by the assessors.

Whichever means of assessment is used there is a need to look at what is a valid assessment for a nurse?

Activity 26

> Which of the following would you say is a valid assessment for
> a nurse?
>
> - aseptic technique
> - first aid skills or
>   knowledge
>
> - drug round
> - physical fitness
>
> - communication skills

There is no easy answer to this question except to say that with the
complexity of nursing there must be a multitude of assessment tools
and assessment situations.

With the multitude of assessment situations there must be
appropriate assessment tools. However, it may be questioned as to
whether an assessment tool is needed to assess what the assessor
should already know and practise.

Activity 27

> Consider the following scenario and decide whether you agree
> with it or not.

Scenario 9

> During a teaching session one day a qualified nurse on a teaching and
> assessing course was asked to design an assessment tool to assess a
> student nurse performing an injection. The qualified nurse stated that
> she did not see the need for writing out an assessment tool. Her
> statement was based on her judgement that she was correct in her
> assessment of students in this situation. She taught the student
> nurse, then let the student nurse practise. Afterwards, she said
> whether the student nurse performed appropriately or not. So, why
> have an assessment tool?

Stenhouse (1975) may support the qualified nurse mentioned in
scenario 9 in this opinion, although the statement concerns the teacher.
'The teacher, as an expert in nursing, can judge the quality of what is
observed without having to define what the quality might consist of in
advance.'

This questions the need for an assessment tool as the qualified nurse
should also be the expert in nursing practice.

Coates and Chambers (1992) state that, 'suitable instruments are
difficult to locate, and also to design.'

However, reliability between assessors will be threatened if there
are no generally agreed criteria concerning appropriate quality.

The next section will critically look at assessment tools.

How can assessment be made reliable?

The answer to this must be twofold.

* The assessment criteria must be clear.
* The assessor and assessee must understand the expectations of the assessment and the related criteria.

The assessment criteria are found within the assessment tool.
The component parts of an assessment tool fall into two areas :

i) Aspects to be looked for — breadth
The aspects to be looked for can appear in statements such as learning outcomes, standards, competencies or in described observable behaviour.

ii) Criteria as to the expected level — depth
The level to be achieved comes in the form of a pass/fail criterion.

The following are a few examples of assessment tools that may be used in clinical practice. The tools are presented, as tables, with comments regarding possible difficulties in use.

The following tools are designed to look at an aspect of patient care.

Activity 28

Look at the following tables and decide whether the tool allows for both breadth and depth, areas i) and ii) as identified earlier.

Assessment tool

Routine admission of a patient

Table 1a

The satisfactory nurse	Tick
Prepares the patient's bed in advance	
Meets patient (and companion) and introduces self	
Establishes a rapport with patient	
Shows the patient his bed area	
Ensures privacy while the patient is unpacking and changing	
Introduces the patient to other patients	
Orientates patient to the clinical area	
Gives appropriate initial information	
Allows the patient to ask questions	
Makes an arrangement for further explanation and discussion	
Demonstrates the appropriate procedures with regard to patient's property	

Table 1b

The unsatisfactory nurse	Tick
Is not prepared for the patient	
Does not welcome the patient	
Does not reassure the patient	
Is formal, abrupt, rushed during the admission procedure	
Omits provision of amenities, eg. jug of water	
Overloads patient with detailed explanations	
Does not orientate patient	

The assessment form (*Tables 1a and b*) allows for a tick system on observed behaviour whether the behaviour is satisfactory or unsatisfactory. However, it does not give a clear indication of what constitutes a pass. It also leaves a question with regard to how many ticks in the unsatisfactory column constitute a fail.

Another assessment form may use a numerical scale or grading scale. The student is given a score from 1 to 6 depending whether s/he is good or poor (1 = poor, 6 = good).

Table 2

Scores	1	2	3	4	5	6
Prepares the patient's bed area in advance						
Meets patient (and companion) and introduces self						
Establishes a rapport with patient						
Shows the patient his bed area						
Ensures privacy while the patient is unpacking and changing						
Introduces patient to other patients						
Orientates patient to the clinical area						
Gives appropriate initial information						
Allows the patient to ask questions						
Makes an arrangement for further explanation and discussion						
Demonstrates the appropriate procedures with regard to patient's property						

This assessment tool still raises questions as to what exactly the student has to do to achieve a pass while additionally raising questions as to what constitutes a score of, for example, 2, 3, or 4 on each aspect.

Take, for example, a situation of assessment related to the process of handwashing, an important aspect of nursing.

If handwashing was graded in six categories what would be satisfactory?

Table 2b

	1	2	3	4	5	6
Washes hands according to procedure						

If 6 = good, then 4, 5 and 6 could be a pass. However what does the student have to do to obtain a pass?

* If the hand washing procedure consisted of 6 stages then possibly the student needs to complete 4, 5 or 6 of the stages to pass. Is this acceptable?
* Also, if the stages are not completed in the order of the procedure although 4, 5 or 6 stages were completed would that matter?

Descriptive rating scales are another form of assessment tool.

The admission procedure could be assessed by using the following performance rating scale.

Table 3

	Performance levels
6	Can perform this skill competently
5	Can perform this skill satisfactorily with initiative and adaptability to problem situations
4	Can perform this skill satisfactorily without assistance and/or supervision
3	Can perform this skill satisfactorily but requires periodic assistance and/or supervision
2	Can perform parts of this skill satisfactorily but requires considerable assistance and/or supervision
1	Has some knowledge about this skill but cannot perform the skill satisfactorily

This assessment tool allows the assessor to expect the student to fail if they award a score of 1 but, in fact, the student could fail with a score of 3 depending on the stage in the course and the level of skill attainment that should be achieved.

Steinaker and Bell (1979) identify five levels of skill acquisition that can be used for assessment. These are: exposure, participation, identification, internalisation and dissemination.

It is important that the assessor actually knows what each of these levels means if they are the criteria of assessment.

The following is an example of the application of the theory of Steinaker and Bell (1979) to the situation of learning to drive a car.

Exposure: At this stage the learner is sitting in the passenger seat observing the driver.

Participation: The first driving lesson and subsequent lessons when the learner is being given detailed guidance. In other words, step by step instructions. For example, put the key in the ignition, check the gears, turn the engine on.

Identification: The learner is now able to complete parts of the skill independently and only requires some further guidance, such as look in your mirror before you pull out.

Internalisation: The stage when the learner is able to perform the actual skill without any need for guidance. The learner is also able to justify his/her actions. At this stage in learning to drive, the instructor is only giving the learner directions to take on the road, no actual guidance is given and the learner should be ready to take the driving test.

Dissemination: The stage when the learner has successfully passed his/her driving test and is now the instructor.

Activity 29

Link the theory of Steinaker and Bell to the learning of a skill in your clinical area.

The following is an example of the theory of Steinaker and Bell applied to the situation where the student has to achieve the competence of 'giving health education to a patient'. The example includes the actions of the mentor/assessor in ensuring that the competence is achieved safely for the patient.

Exposure: The student observes the mentor/assessor giving health education to a patient.

Participation: The student is instructed by the mentor/assessor as to his/her actions. The actions are justified.

Identification: The student is asked to discuss the health education needs of a patient, identifying and discussing with rationale the education to be given with their mentor/ assessor. At this stage the mentor/assessor is required to give some guidance and advice.

Internalisation: The student can now give the health education required for a patient with justification. This stage again can occur between the mentor/assessor and the student without the patient present. At this stage the mentor/ assessor can ensure as much as possible that the student is capable of giving the accurate information to a patient.

Dissemination: The student can now give health education directly to the patient under the supervision of the mentor/assessor initially, until assessed as competent.

An understanding of the theory of Steinaker and Bell links to the assessment form in that each statement on an assessment form needs to be closely regarded and accurately comprehended by the assessor and the assessee.

Take, for example, the UKCC Code of Professional Conduct statement:

no action or omission on your part, or within your sphere of responsibility, is detrimental to the interests, condition or safety of patients and clients.

This has been discussed with regard to the interpretation of punctuality and attendance on *page 46*. If the assessors are not in agreement concerning the meaning of the statements/criteria on an assessment form then there will be unreliability of assessment.

In some instances, according to Steinaker and Bell (1979), the assessor need not know which level the student has to achieve to pass. Not knowing the level to be achieved could mean that the assessor judges on demonstrated behaviour and avoids the error of leniency or the error of severity — see *page 73*.

Assessment using outcomes or competence statements

Benner (1984) identifies the competent stage. Statements of competence have been made on many assessment forms and the student's achievement has been identified through use of criteria such as Steinaker and Bell (1979) or through production of evidence.

The following are two examples:
1. Competence
    An end competence statement: The student should be able to assess patients within the acute clinical area.
    One element of competence: The student can identify and apply the skills required in assessment.

Exposure	Participation	Identification	Internalisation	Dissemination
Observe action	Work under instruction	Work with part instruction	Work without instruction	Work and teach others

The **evidence** would take the form of either a verbal description and/or demonstration of the admission skills required; **and/or** a written description of the admission skills required.

This means of assessment raises some difficulty of interpretation as the assessor needs to be clear concerning the number of skills required and the breadth and depth of knowledge required of the student to achieve a satisfactory level.

2.   Competence
An end competence statement: The student should be able to demonstrate proficient nursing intervention in the clinical area..
Element of competence: The student should be able to discuss the managerial and clinical factors that influence the safety of the clinical area.

This competence raises some essential questions and cannot be seen in isolation.

In order to complete this competence for a student the assessor needs to know:

- level/stage of training
- expected level of knowledge
- level of knowledge to be achieved.

Looking just at the factors that influence safety could give rise to a long list of policies/procedures, of which the following are only a few:

- fire procedure
- health and safety regulations
- control of infections policy
- manual handling policy
- COSHH

If these policies/procedures are identified how many and to what depth does the student need to demonstrate knowledge?

For example, with the fire procedure should the student be able to state:

I.   Action to be taken on hearing the alarm bell
   * respond
   * ensure one person has gone to the fire point
   * close doors and windows
   * ensure patients are safe.

II. Identify where the alarm button/s are in the area.

III. State where the fire hose and extinguishers are kept.

IV. Describe how an electrical fire would be handled.

Using Steinaker and Bell in this instance might be problematic, eg. exposure/participation. The exposure should come in the initial explanation and introduction to the ward; participation and identification should come on questioning in the interim period.

However, how much should the student know to be competent?

If all aspects apart from 'ensure one person has gone to the fire point' are answered correctly, should the competence be signed?

Critical areas of assessment need to be identified.

A competence statement is a broad outline; an assessor needs to identify the specifics. Butterworth (1996) advocates that assessors need a shared set of standards.

As a broad outline this competence raises other problems, ie. that of time. How long will it take to discuss the policies/procedures related to maintaining a safe environment? It's like asking the question, 'How long is a piece of string?' Is it sufficient that the student knows where the policy/procedure documents are kept? This would certainly need less time than a discussion on the actual procedure.

It would appear that staff in a clinical area would need to identify the specifics of competence statements completed in their area to give some reliability to assessment. Students would need to be informed of these specifics during the introduction to the clinical area.

Activity 30

> Discuss with colleagues in your clinical area the specific expectations for the following competence for a student on placement in your clinical area.
>
> Identify the communication systems used within the clinical area and evaluate their effectiveness.

Discussion with colleagues may highlight various subjective opinions but should lead to a consensus and an objective set of specific statements and criteria related to the competence statement.

Conclusion

At the end of this section the reader should be able to:
- describe a valid assessment situation for a nurse
- state a means of making an assessment reliable
- justify responses to the following situations:
    * Jessica asks for guidance on how to communicate satisfactorily with patients in order to achieve an A, B, or C grade on her report.
    * Danny feels that nursing is all practical work and, unless he is doing his mental health allocation, does not feel that he needs assessment of his communication skills. Besides, he has a degree in psychology so probably knows more than you do.

References and suggested further reading

Apgar V (1953) A proposal for a new method of evaluation of the new-born infant. *Curr Res Anaesthesia and Analgesia* **32**: 253–267

Apgar V (1953) Care of the Neonate. Cited in: Carter B (ed) (1993) *Manual of Paediatric Intensive Care Nursing.* Chapman and Hall, London: ch 3

Beaumont G (1996) Review of 100 NVQ's and SVQ's. NCVQ/SCOTVEC CAEL (1975) CAEL Working Paper No 6. *A Guide for Assessing Prior Experience through Portfolios, Cooperative Assessment of Experiential Learning.* Educational Testing Service, USA

Benner P (1984) *From Novice to Expert: Excellence and Power in Clinical Nursing Practice.* Addison Wesley, California

Butterworth C (1996) Going soft on Assessment. *New Academic* **5**(1): 12–13

Clifford C (1994) Assessment of Clinical Practice and the Role of the Nurse Teacher. *Nurse Ed Today* **14**: 272–279

Coates VE, Chambers M (1992) Evaluation of tools to assess clinical competence. *Nurse Ed Today* **12**: 122–129

College of Occupational Therapists (1989–1991) An Introduction for Health Care Professionals. Cited in: Wright CC, Whittington D (1992) *Quality Assurance.* Churchill Livingstone, Edinburgh

Cotton J (1995)*The Theory of Assessment. An Introduction.* Kogan Page, London

Further Education Curriculum Unit (1984) *Towards a Competency-based System.* FEU, London

Jarvis P, Gibson S (1997) *The Teacher Practitioner in Nursing, Midwifery, Health Visiting and the Social Services*, 2nd edn. Stanley Thornes, Cornwall

Norton D (1975) *An investigation of geriatric problems in hospital.* Churchill Livingstone, Edinburgh

Oppenheim AN (1984) *Questionnaire Design and Attitude Measurement.* Heinemann, London

Purdy M (1997) *The problem of self-assessment in nurse education.* Nurse Ed Today 17: 135–139

Quinn FM (1995) *Principles and Practice of Nurse Education*, 3rd edn. Chapman Hall, London

Ross M, Carroll G, Knight J *et al* (1988) Using the OSCE to measure clinical skills performance in nursing. *J Adv Nurs* **13**: 45–56

Rowntree D (1987) *Assessing Students: How shall we know them?* Kogan Page, London

Steinaker NW, Bell MR (1979) *The Experimental Taxonomy.* Academic Press, New York

Stengelhofen J (1993) *Teaching Students in Clinical settings.* Chapman and Hall, London

Stenhouse L (1975) *Introduction to Curriculum Research and Development.* Heinemann, London

United Kingdom Central Council (1992) *The Code of Professional Conduct.* UKCC, London

Waterlow JA (1985) A risk assessment card. *Nurs Times* **81**(48): 49–55

Waterlow JA (1996) Pressure sore assessments. *Nurs Times* **92**(29): 53–58

Wright CC, Whittington D (1992) *Quality Assurance. An Introduction for Health Care Professionals.* Churchill Livingstone, Edinburgh

6

The role of the assessor

Assessment can affect people in a variety of ways.

Activity 31

Recall your feelings when being assessed in the past.

You may say that you felt stress, anxiety, worry and/or fear; you may even have felt physical effects such as shaking, sweating and trembling or less frequently nausea or frequency of micturition.

A certain level of stress is beneficial to performance levels but too much stress can hinder performance levels.

Part of the assessor's role is to reduce stress for the student.

It also needs to be remembered that the assessor can be subject to stress. Stress for the assessor can come from many different sources but the assessor has to learn to cope with these stresses of assessment.

Stresses related to assessment could include the:

- number of assessments that have to be completed
- repetition of assessment
- fatigue associated with assessment
- boredom of assessment
- emotional, conscience-searching aspects of the responsibility of passing or failing a student.

This chapter will concentrate on the role, functions and qualities of the assessor in an assessment situation that has been pre-arranged. This situation may occur as part of continuous assessment of practice or as a separate entity.

Role of assessor

The role of the assessor in the clinical area is twofold.

It includes the function of assessment and also the important function of maintaining safety and standards.

Everett (1995) states that 'the assessor is accountable both to the learner in giving a fair judgement and to the public in ensuring the standards of professional competence are achieved'.

MacGuire (1984) states that 'the good assessor needs not only to be able to judge performance in an unbiased way, but to maximise the chances of reaching the required standard by paying attention to all the apparently extraneous elements that help make or mar an assessment'.

The assessor is ultimately responsible for the safety of the situation and this means that she, or a named substitute, must be present for the duration of the assessment. It may also mean that she might need to take some action to ensure the safety of the situation.

Assessment periods may vary in length and there appears to be no agreed time, interval or period set for the performance of continuous assessment. The choice of the substitute(s) is important. A substitute is most likely in continuous assessment.

The assessor in the pre-arranged situation

How can safety be maintained?

The following are a series of actions that the assessor can make to ensure a safe situation prior to the commencement of the assessment.

Discuss the assessment requirements with the student

If the student knows what is expected then s/he will stand a better chance of handling the situation him/herself. Knowing the expectation is a requirement, it may also lower the anxiety level of the student.

The student may request a 'trial run', a formative practice that may be with the assessor or another member of qualified staff. The trial run may allow for some potentially unsafe issues to be addressed.

Ensure that the student is able to undertake the assessment on the day

This involves the assessor in ensuring that the student is in a fit state both physically and mentally to undertake the assessment. It may be a difficult decision as the anxiety of assessment can make some students very unwell. However, due to the fact that a variety of reasons may render the student unable to take the assessment as arranged, the assessor should always make a point of asking the student if s/he is ready to commence the assessment.

All policies linked to assessment have a section concerning extenuating circumstances. This means that the student can, within the guidelines of the policy, raise issues that have resulted in poor performance. The assessor needs to have asked the student if these circumstances exist before the assessment commences so that appropriate action can be taken and neither the assessor nor the student will spend the time of assessment unnecessarily.

Even with these actions taken an assessment may still raise issues of safety. Therefore, the assessor must consider **when and whether she needs to take action during an assessment**.

It must be noted that if an assessor has to take action during an assessment to make the situation safe then the student performance for this assessment is not considered to be satisfactory.

Aspects to consider during an assessment if a situation becomes unsafe:

- whether the assessor's intervention needs to be immediate. The assessor may allow the student appropriate time to make the situation safe
- whether the assessment should stop when the assessor takes action
- whether, in all instances, the student needs to know that the assessor has taken action.

Stopping the assessment may depend on the effect that the assessor's action has on the student. It is worth considering turning the assessment into a teaching session if the student realises s/he has made a mistake and consequently loses confidence.

Allowing the student to finish the assessment may allow for restoration of that confidence.

The assessor's actions during an assessment

If the assessor takes action during an assessment then there may be two reasons:

1. As mentioned above it is as a reaction to ensure safety in a situation.
2. It may be by prior arrangement before the assessment started that the assessor could be asked to assist where needed. If this is the case the assessor must remember to follow instructions and the student must be informed before the assessment that clear instructions must be given to the assessor. If this is not the case, then the assessor may end up leading the student's actions or even be in conflict with the student's intentions.

The assessor also needs to inform the student of what might happen during the assessment. This can include writing notes or re-positioning to see and hear more clearly and, therefore, the student need not be concerned with what the assessor is doing but should concentrate on the task in hand.

The student need not treat the assessor as a guest in the situation. The student does not have to introduce the assessor to the patient/s involved in the assessment. The involvement and permission seeking from patients needs to be clarified between the student and the assessor before the assessment.

In some instances the assessor will have to decide which patient/s will be involved in the assessment and then ask the patient's permission. Where possible, the assessor will then notify the student.

In other instances the student may decide on the patient and the assessor will then introduce herself to the patient and ask permission for the assessment to commence.

On occasions the student may decide on the patient and ask him for permission and then either introduce the assessor or not.

Whichever is the approach to be taken, the assessor and student must agree.

In a continuous assessment situation, both the student and the assessor may be known to the patient and the issue of permission is unlikely to arise.

The choice of patients to allow for assessment situations can raise some difficulties. This situation may not be realistic due to the turnover of patients.

Selecting a patient before an assessment and informing the student of the selection can create a problem related to the fact that the student will especially rehearse for the one situation. This rehearsal could compromise the student's adaptability to any situation, and the need to assess that skill.

Other problems may arise from the changes in the patient's condition from the time of selection until the time of assessment. Change in a patient's condition could be either an improvement or a deterioration. An improvement in a patient's condition may mean then that the student is not being adequately tested. A deterioration may, in some instances, mean that the student is to be required to perform skills outside of his/her expected level of knowledge and skills. There may be some assessment situations where the student would still be expected to act safely and seek appropriate assistance in the care of a patient whose condition has deteriorated.

Further considerations that the assessor may have to make concern the following situations:

i.   The student is not happy with the skills required to nurse the selected patient/s.
ii.   The patient's condition changes during the assessment period.
iii.   The patient feels that he is being assessed as well.
iv.   The assessor avoiding being influenced by the feelings of the patient for the nurse, eg. 'halo effect'.

Situation i):   This should be avoided by correct decision-making by the assessor. If the situation does occur after the decision then the assessor must review the patient and decide that the skills required of the student are actually realistic for him/her to achieve. This action should prevent the student from being able to manipulate a situation to make assessment easier.

Situation ii):   The assessor must quickly review the situation and ensure that the newly required skills for the patient's care are within the remit of the student. If new actions have to be taken then the assessor must take action and inform the student accordingly. The assessor's action in this instance should not affect the assessment result.

Situation iii):   The assessor may have spoken to individual patients involved in the assessment and explained the role of the patient where necessary. However, the assessor needs to be aware of the possible 'Hawthorne effect' (Handy, 1985), that is the potential effect on a patient's behaviour of being paid an exceptional amount of attention.

Situation iv):   The assessor needs to remain objective although valuing the patient's opinion if given.

Other considerations:

- remember to give the student some personal space — the assessor does not need, in all instances, to peer over his/her shoulder
- the assessor's use of verbal and non-verbal cues during an assessment.

Activity 32

> Make a list of the types of non-verbal communication that may occur during an assessment. Consider how these may be: a) misunderstood or b) minimised.

Non-verbal cues can include posture, movement, writing and facial expressions, such as a smile or a grimace. A smile or a grimace may convey the wrong meaning so beware. Smiling all the time is inappropriate, so remain detached. Breathing, too, eg. sighing, yawning, gasping, even quietly can give distinct messages to students.

Verbal communication during an assessment can be off-putting, especially if the assessor asks a question that the student cannot answer or only partly answer. Questions need to be appropriate and asked at the appropriate time.

They must also have a relevance to the assessment situation. If the student is asked a question the assessor must know what is expected as an answer. Also, if the student answers incorrectly or only partly the assessor must be aware of the effect that this will have on the assessment outcome.

So, remember, questions should not be indiscriminate.

Appropriate times to question a student during an assessment:

* At the commencement of the assessment to ensure that the student is ready and able to start.

* During an assessment if the assessor wishes to determine what the student is intending to do next. For example, as already mentioned, the assessor does not need to look over the student's shoulder all the time; it may be important for the patient to be allowed rest periods so the assessor may question when the student next intends to give care to the patient. This may give rise to a situation when the assessor does not have to be present for the duration of the assessment if the student is looking after other patients not involved in the assessment situation. The assessor may then agree on a time to return to the assessment.

The assessor needs to consider, when asking the student what s/he intends to do next, that the student is not being prompted into action, for example, if the assessor asked the student: 'When are you going to be giving Mr X his drugs?' This is a loaded or prompting question.

It is not considered appropriate to question students during the performance of a skill as this may mean that the student stops in order to answer the question and this may then lead to loss of concentration and disrupt the skilled procedure under observation.

Bloom's taxonomy of psychomotor skills (1956) identifies a level of performance of a skill with incorporation of other skills which include verbalisation. Levels of skill acquisition according to Bloom are:

Limitation: when a skill is observed and copied
Manipulation: when a skill is performed according to instruction rather than observation.
Precision: when a skill is performed accurately without instruction
Articulation: when an original skill is performed with other skills at a similar time. For example, the skill of driving combined with the skill of talking either to a passenger or on a mobile phone. It should be noted at this point that some skills do not go well in combination, for

example, the use of a mobile phone while driving. This is now strongly discouraged by the police. Articulation also means that the skill can be talked about while it is being performed, ie. doing the skill while reflecting on it. It can also mean questioning at the end of the assessment or during the feedback process.

Naturalisation: one or more skills are performed with ease as they have become automatic. For example, bathing a patient, observing the state of their skin and talking to him at the same time, while instructing a junior member of staff in the patient's care as well.

Remember the intended level of assessment. For example, if an assessment involves only the level of manipulation, the student should be assessed only on this, not on a higher level of skill such as precision or articulation.

Questions during an assessment can also unsettle the student if s/he is unsure of the answer. However, to ensure safety of the situation the assessor may have to question a student on an intended action. Take, for example, the situation of needing to call relatives in to see a patient who has deteriorated. It may not be safe to allow the student to go and pick up the phone and call the relatives without the assessor finding out first what the student intends to say to the relatives.

This may avoid situations such as the following. During an assessment a student phoned relatives and said, 'xxxx's blood pressure is very high and he has not had a good night. He is not feeling very well and neither is he looking very well. You had better come and visit.'

On putting the phone down the student remarked, 'I do not know why the relatives always get upset when I phone them.'

Clearly, this student needed formative help in relation to this aspect of care.

Psychological considerations

This next section will look in more detail at some of the psychological considerations before discussing giving feedback.

Activity 33

Consider how you, as an assessor, can help reduce stress: i) in the student and ii) in yourself.

Here is a list of possible solutions or suggestions to help reduce stress in the student:

> be approachable
>
> give clear explanations
>
> be careful of non-verbal cues
>
> consider verbal communication.

Here is a list of possible solutions or suggestions for helping reduce stress as an assessor:

> be on time
>
> have no other commitments for the assessment period, eg. being 'in charge' of the ward
>
> ensure ability to see and hear throughout the assessment
>
> if possible avoid fatigue — early nights, good diet, exercise
>
> create a support system with colleagues to discuss thoughts and feelings confidentially if needed, and to ensure consistency
>
> ensure reliability of mentoring/assessing with knowledge of the assessment format
>
> ensure understanding of the assessment criteria.

Criteria for assessment are important, they should help to reduce bias and subjectivity by the assessor. Subjectivity is one of the biggest problems of assessment; bias may be denied but is this true?

Activity 34

Make a list of the personal attributes/characteristics that you find in individuals:
■ pleasing ■ irritating
List the personal attributes/characteristics that are unique to you that others may find:
■ pleasing ■ irritating

As an assessor be aware that:

- prejudices can influence an assessor
- potential prejudices of a student may influence the perceptions of the assessor.

An assessor needs to raise her level of awareness by thinking through potential influences/prejudices, as these can often be the aspects that cause stress for the assessor.

Take, for example, the student who is spoken about with high regard by patients and other members of staff. Will this not influence the assessor's view as to how the student will perform even before the assessment commences?

Likewise, the student who is liked by the patients but unpopular with other members of staff as too much time is spent talking to the patients and not helping with the work.

Other factors to consider are:

'Halo effect': The halo effect can have a positive or negative influence on the assessor's opinion, eg. the tendency for the glowing report to prejudice the assessor in favour of the student, and the tendency for previous negative assessments to bias the assessor against the student.

Often the comment on report forms is 'nice nurse should do well'. It is questionable whether this comment has been written with regard to the nurse's standard of work or the fact that they get on well with the assessor.

Error of leniency: Being too lenient or overlooking errors which require attention. This can occur if, for any reason, the assessor is over concerned about the student or about her own response to the student.

For example, knowledge of the anxiety state of the student in the assessment process might sway the assessor to allow an action due to nervousness. It is easier to be kind in these situations.

Error of severity: This is an error in the opposite direction to the error of leniency, made for similar but opposite reasons. For example, the assessor may be unhappy with the attitude of a student and take particular exception to a comment made and possibly look for subsequent errors to enable failure of the student. Alternatively, an assessor may feel no student is very good and always give low marks.

If an assessor recognises that they personally have a bias concerning the student, either that they like or they dislike them, then the error of leniency or the error of severity may be employed. It is not always that the 'dislike' bias will indicate the error of severity or that the 'like' bias would indicate the error of leniency. There may be the instance when the assessor 'likes' the student but wants them to do exceptionally well, especially when they have taught/mentored the student and, therefore, may be exceptionally critical. In either instance, there can also be an overcompensation which may influence the expectations and the result of the assessment.

Central tendency: Often in this instance the assessor is not very pleased with the student's performance or not concerned either way. The easier option is to mark the middle grade if there is one. This allows the student to pass but does not really give a good reflection of performance. It is also what happens if a test is not discriminating well or if the assessor is wary of giving extreme grades.

Activity 35

> Identify instances from your own experience that would equate with the halo effect, an error of leniency and/or an error of severity.
> List the factors that may have influenced the assessor in the instances identified.
> Identify the factors that may influence your judgement as an assessor.

The assessor's role in the assessment feedback

Whichever type of assessment is completed, part of the role of the assessor is to report back to the student on his/her performance.

The next section will look at this aspect.

Activity 36

> Think about an assessment situation when a student did not do well. How would you convey the result?

In giving assessment feedback the assessor needs to think about several issues. These issues can be linked to the theory of Maslow (1971).

Physical needs

Assessment periods vary and it can be that feedback is being given at the end of a shift. This may mean that the student and assessor are tired or hungry, so consider when the student can best be given the feedback. It is not possible to give a definitive answer as each situation will vary. The apprehension of the student for his/her feedback may mean that s/he does not want to eat anyway. However, if the discussion following the assessment is liable to be lengthy then the assessor may have to make the decision for the student. Also, consider elimination needs: anxiety can create frequency of micturition so it is worth asking the student if s/he is ready for her results/placement feedback.

Safety needs

Assessment feedback is very personal to the student so the student must feel secure in the fact that s/he is going to be told this first. It is important to consider the environment to allow the student safety and privacy and uninterrupted time to assimilate the assessment result and the accompanying feedback. Assessment feedback can sometimes be similar to situations of giving patients or relatives bad news. This may mean that the student becomes very distressed. Even giving surprisingly good results can produce distress-like reactions as the anxiety and relief that the student experiences may produce an 'hysterical', tearful, demonstrative response. Whatever the result the student is going to receive, it is advisable to prepare each feedback environment in the same way:

- allow the student to sit at the same level as the assessor
- arrange the chairs so that there is personal space but that they are partly facing, at a 90-degree angle
- make sure that the student is sitting away from the door. There may be instances when the student is distressed by the results and may want to rush from the room in this distressed state. Leaving the room may mean that the student is then in the view of other staff or patients when s/he may be verbally or emotionally upset. The student needs protection at this time until s/he can cope with the results; therefore, it is better to keep him/her in the room until s/he has been able to express either tearfully or angrily his/her distress.

The assessor may need at this time to take on a 'counselling' role.

Belonging and love

Whatever the result of the placement assessment the student needs to feel involved. The assessee's opinion and views on the assessment process need to be expressed. In most instances, this can be done by the assessor first asking the assessee, 'How do you feel that you have done?'

However, the assessor may question whether the student should be told immediately by the assessor if s/he has passed or not.

There is no clear-cut answer to each situation. It is suggested that the student is asked how s/he has done on first or formative attempts at an assessment. On a final or summative attempt at an assessment, when consequences may be severe, the student needs to know initially whether s/he has passed or failed. Asking the student about the assessment allows for self-assessment and involves the process of reflection; both of these approaches are seen as a means of learning. This illustrates the point that assessments are also learning periods.

Purdy (1997) states that 'self-assessment may provide the subjective component which makes the teacher's objective observations of the student more accurate and complete'. However, Purdy goes further to say that 'nurse education emphasises professional selection at the expense of personal, professional development'.

Kenworthy and Nicklin (1989) state that self-assessment produces 'flexible practitioners engaged in a future of life-long learning'.

It is worth considering whether a student who, at the end of an assessment, cannot identify whether s/he has given safe care should be allowed to give any care in an unsupervised manner?

Boud (1991) states that,

Self-assessment requires the students to think critically about what they are learning, to identify appropriate standards of performance and to apply them to their own work. Self-assessment encourages students to look to themselves and to other sources to determine what criteria should be used in judging their work rather than being dependent solely on their teachers or other authorities.

Reflective practice has been advocated for some time (Schon, 1983). Reflection is seen as an essential part of the learning process because it results in making sense of, or extracting meaning from, the experience (Osterman, 1990). Reflection involves thinking about and critically analysing actions with the purpose of improving professional practice. The assessee may need help with the process of reflection.

Dunn (1991) has suggested that 'validity and reliability would be enhanced if student nurses assessed their own learning'. When asked how s/he has performed s/he may often be very self-critical. After a written examination students are heard to say, 'Oh I have failed that'. Likewise, students assessed in practice may say, 'I have not done very well'. This is not the time for the assessor to give the verdict on the assessment but the time for the assessor to allow further reflection by asking the student why s/he thinks s/he has not done well. It is also the approach an assessor can take when the student says s/he has done all right whether s/he has or not. What has occurred during the time of the assessment can be discussed. The assessor can ask the student to say whether s/he would have handled any instance differently if it occurred again or the student can be asked to justify his/her actions during the assessment. While this discussion is going on and before the student has been told the result of the assessment, positive aspects of performance can be discussed along with negative aspects if they have occurred. It is hoped that during this discussion the student will become more aware of his/her actions and recognition of good performance will give him/her more confidence and negative actions can be corrected.

Esteem needs

Discussing the assessment with the student should help his/her self-esteem. It is often better for students to hear positive points first but it is also important to leave the student with some positive aspects. Again, there is no hard and fast rule with regard to the order of feedback but it is worth bearing in mind that once the assessor has given a decision the student's participation in the learning process will diminish either from relief or distress.

A fairly helpful rubric for the assessor when giving feedback is to make a positive overall comment first, then to consider specific points in detail and to finish with a positive overall comment.

Self-actualisation

Positive assessment results help achievement and the process of self-actualisation but negative results can also be looked on as a positive means of assisting in self-actualisation. A negative assessment result may help the student to focus his/her thoughts about work/life. This may mean that a career of nursing is more determinedly pursued or that another more suitable career is chosen. The assessor may be involved in helping the student to achieve in nursing by being supportive, offering practical help and guidance towards future assessments or retaking of assessments.

One of the authors recalls a situation where a first year student was given a rather long account by the ward sister of how badly she was performing. Due to the negativity of the sister's comments the student stated that she might as well give up nursing if that was the opinion. The response of the sister to this comment illustrates how vital assessment feedback is and what an important part of learning it can be. The sister said, 'Now, If I did not think you were worth it I would not have bothered to take this time to point out the problems.'

Assessment feedback should make the assessee feel valued and important. If it does, then it will increase self-esteem and ultimately help towards a greater realisation of potential or self-actualisation.

Warrenden (1990) states that 'the most effective way of helping healthcare students to progress towards professional competence is through the provision of clear and regular feedback'.

A final important point on feedback is that it must be objective and should state what happened or what did not happen.

The assessor's word is final with regard to what has occurred or not occurred during a practical assessment. So the assessor must be sure of what she saw or heard or did not see or hear.

The assessor needs a clear conscience that she has given a fair result. This clear conscience can be based on actual occurrences or omissions during the assessment period. Giving a positive assessment result is nice for an assessor but, in the instances of giving a negative result, the assessor, as well as the student, may feel emotionally distressed. Being sure of the assessment decision can alleviate some of the distress but the effect on the student and his/her continuation of training can often affect the assessor. It is worth having a support system, for example, a colleague or clinical supervisor or superior to discuss the assessment with if necessary. This discussion can be done confidentially and the student's name need not be mentioned but the circumstances of the assessment may be reviewed. This sort of discussion can reinforce for the assessor the fact that she made the correct decision. Assessment does make an assessor question her beliefs, values, expectations and standards by reflection on the assessment process.

Conclusion

At the end of this section the reader should be able to:
- identify his/her own feelings with regard to assessment
- state and critically compare expected performance outcomes concerning one clinical action with a colleague
- consider responses to the following situations:

  * Jessica asks why she has to be assessed when it makes her feel so nervous that she cannot sleep or eat properly and feels sick.

  * Danny has asked you out for a drink even though he knows you are responsible for the completion of his assessment document.

References and suggested reading

Bloom B (1956) *Taxonomy of Educational Objectives: The Classification of Educational Goals. Handbook One: Cognitive Domain.* McKay, New York

Boud D (1991) *Implementing Student Self-Assessment,* 2nd edn. Kogan Page, London

Dunn B (1991) A caring curriculum. *Senior Nurse* **11**(6): 12–15

Everett A (1995) The educational role of the community mental health nurse. *Ment Health Nurs* **15**(9): 8–10

Handy CB (1985) *Understanding Organisations.* Penguin, London

Kenworthy N, Nicklin P (1989) *Teaching and Assessing in Nursing Practice. An experiential approach.* Scutari, London

MacGuire J (1984) Assessing the assessor. *Senior Nurse* **9**(1): 12–13

Maslow A (1971) *The Farther Reaches of Human Nature.* Penguin, Harmondsworth

Osterman KF (1990) Reflective Practice: A New Agenda for Education. *Education and Urban Society* **22**(2): 133–152

Purdy M (1997) The problem of self-assessment in nurse education. *Nurse Ed Today* **17**: 135–139

Rowntree D (1987) *Assessing Students: How shall we know them?* Kogan Page, London

Schon D (1983) *The Reflective Practitioner.* Basic Books, New York

Warrendon F (1990) Clinical Practice. A student centred learning package. *Br J Occ Ther* **53**(6): 233–238

7

Forms of assessment

The following chapter will discuss:
i)   Prearranged assessments
ii) Continuous assessment
iii) Objective structured clinical assessment
iv) Accreditation of prior learning AP(E)L.

Individual practical assessments have been described by Kenworthy and Nicklin (1989) as a series of 'snapshots' of a student's performance. They suggest that photographs can be taken by a variety of people, including the student, to gain a wide picture of the level of performance. Perhaps continuous practical assessment could be likened to closed circuit television which is consistently recording but not necessarily viewed in entirety but aspects are highlighted when something different — good or bad — occurs. This could mean that continuous assessment is a mixture of 'snapshots' and overall performance of a student.

Whichever form of assessment is used, assessment needs to be based on specific evidence rather than intuitive thinking. Girot (1993) comments on intuitive thinking stating that those who assess clinical competencies operate at an intuitive level rather than with specific evidence. It is questionable whether the intuitive approach is valid and/or reliable. Intuition could operate on the basis of knowledge or it could be more superficial and dependent on the assessor's mood and temper on a particular day or the personality chemistry between student and assessor.

Benner (1984) and Schon (1983), who are well known for their focus on reflective practice, support the use of specific evidence for assessment. This corroborates earlier discussion in *chapter 1* of the need to see and hear what is being assessed.

It could be argued that temperamental factors, attitudes or prejudices (see *chapter 6*) could bias any type of assessment. These factors may be inappropriate in assessment situations. Others involved in the assessment process, eg. the patient, may also create or be subjected to bias. These issues need to be recognised and addressed as they introduce factors which complicate assessment.

The following sections consider how to deal with assessment.

Prearranged assessment

An important question to consider with assessment is whether the student should be informed in advance that s/he is going to be assessed or whether s/he could be assessed and informed of the result on completion of the performance.

Some assessment formats might allow for this warning whereas others do not. Prearranged assessments do allow for this notification. Prearranged assessment has been covered in some detail in *chapter 6*.

Everden (1986) discusses that the artificiality of the single clinical assessment (prearranged assessment) has a potential to compromise standards. The assessment can be rehearsed and as result might not represent a consistent standard of performance by the assessee (Exton and Smith, 1976), neither might the assessment represent future performance and this could compromise validity.

Main points concerning prearranged/one off assessments.The student:

- has notification
- may become more anxious
- can rehearse for the assessment
- may perform for this occasion only.

The assessment may:

- produce a rote learned behaviour rather than understanding or application
- examine only stated aspects
- produce varied assessment situations due to varied patient conditions and changes, therefore causing inconsistency
- allow for a realistic situation
- be influenced by the patient's response to the assessment scenario.

Continuous assessment

In the following discussion on continuous assessment a dual picture will be presented by examining the advantages and disadvantages of continuous assessment.

Continuous assessment according to the ENB (1996) is 'a series of progressively updated measurements of a student's achievement and progress'.

Clifford (1994) states that 'continuous practical assessment implies that student performance is monitored continuously during the day-to-day activities in clinical practice'. Whether the assessment is continuous or spasmodic may vary.

Stoker and Hull (1994) state that 'if a student can do it once its an event, twice may be a coincidence, three times may show a consistent pattern emerging'.

In continuous assessment however a student's skills, knowledge and attitudes should be considered over a specified period of time.

For pre-registration students the measuring tool is normally based on the UKCC Competencies (Rule 18/18A) (see *Appendix*). This assessment can be undertaken by an individual assessor, or a team of assessors.

The purpose of continuous assessment is to assess an individual student's ability on a cumulative basis thus enabling ipsative (see *page 45*) assessment to take place.

Depending on the placement time available, the structure of the process could be:

Introductory assessment

Student self-assessment of learning needs during placement and orientation of student to specific policies, procedures and activities of clinical area.

Midway assessment

This is the time to give the student specific feedback about progress and areas of weakness as matched to the document provided — **formative assessment**.

Final assessment

The document is completed and a discussion should take place giving an opportunity for discussion of gradings awarded — **summative assessment**.

Not all continuous assessment situations can follow the above pattern. Placements, for example, may be too short or too specialised. The structure would then have to be adapted by the university responsible for the student.

The key to continuous practical assessment is good communication over a period of time. It is no use to the student to be told at final assessment that s/he has not fulfilled the set objectives for the placement. Early notification and an agreed plan of action (see learning contracts, *page 40*) are essential to make the process effective.

In continuous assessment variable performance can be viewed over a period of time and, as a result, it may be difficult to determine the final outcome. Conversely a bad day may be overcome by many good days. Had the student been assessed solely on the 'bad day' then the situation would be more difficult to retrieve.

This type of assessment requires close supervision. Often with staff shortages, junior staff nurses unsure of their own roles and over-confident students, it can lead to very arbitrary and patchy assessment.

The student is also working in the real world situation, having to problem solve and work realistically in a team.

Feedback should be given at the point of need. Students also get used to being observed and work more naturally. This enables a truer picture of practice to be seen. The individual student also needs to take responsibility for his/her own learning. What learning strengths and weaknesses does s/he have?

The documents used for assessment are normally geared to the specific experience being assessed. The need to match criteria or specific objectives can mean a lengthy assessment document to complete which is very time consuming. By working with the student over a period of time the assessor may find it difficult to be unbiased. Personality clashes and attractions can influence results.

An advantage of continuous assessment is that standards once achieved can be maintained and improved upon. If a correct procedure is performed it may be difficult to determine whether this level is at academic level 1, 2 or 3. Good practice is good practice. It may be necessary to assess understanding of the practice in a written form or by asking questions to support the level of understanding.

Advantages of continuous assessment:

- snapshots of performance, Kenworthy and Nicklin (1989)
- good/bad and average days viewed
- close supervision
- less threatening situation
- continuous therefore should maintain competence
- real world situation
- problem-solving and therefore linked to the way adults learn, according to Knowles (1984)
- self/personal assessment
- graded to expected level of competence
- continuing set of progressive goals.

Disadvantages of continuous assessment:

- time consuming
- lengthy documents
- shorter clinical placements lead to feedback not being so pertinent
- documents need adapting for different specialities

- questionable generalised suitability
- external factors can affect and influence results, eg. the helpful/ pleasant student , the 'Halo effect'
- can be unreliable and therefore invalid
- personality bias can be either way
- questionable whether different levels of practice can be determined, eg. Level 2 or 3
- volume of students means that all trained staff including most junior may need to assess although they are not experienced
- the assessment is only as good as the assessor
- the student may be viewed as 'coping' and therefore as achieving the assessment
- the student is constantly under scrutiny and so might feel threatened.

Main points of continuous assessment:

- not necessarily prearranged therefore less anxiety provoking
- could lead to surprise assessments
- work with the person who assesses
- can lead to assessor prompting/indicating action
- difficulties related to working with and observing as an assessor at the same time
- should promote consistent standards of performance
- student needs to be observed
- can create bias due to longer periods of contact
- relies on several people as assessors
- creates problems of decisions if performance is variable with both good and bad days.

Prearranged/one off and continuous assessment are not the only means of assessment for nurses. At one time, practical assessment was conducted in a practical room under controlled conditions away from the clinical area.

This next section will looked at a form of assessment that may be conducted in a practical room or within a controlled clinical environment, but with a more 'real life' approach.

Problems of the function, implementation and interpretation of assessment have been mentioned in this book.

Before reading this section complete the following activity.

Activity 37

> List the advantages and disadvantages of current assessment means and tools.

According to Ross *et al* (1988) assessment in clinical practice needs to be thought out; it should not occur by chance with assessee and assessors being unprepared.

The following section will look at a suggestion for assessment of clinical practice that is not altogether new.

Objective structured assessment

Ross (1988) goes further to say that there needs to be:

a method of assessing clinical competence which is objective in nature, fulfilling the criteria of validity, reliability and practicality, with the potential for testing a wide range of knowledge and skills whilst accommodating a large number of examinees.

Activity 35

> Compare the assessment of medical students in practical situations with the ideas of Ross (1988). Think how it would be possible to address the requirements of Ross in your clinical area.

The following is a list of examples of possible situations to consider for the assessment of clinical practice.

These situations can include the assessment of clinical competencies/objectives/learning outcomes. They can be broken down into various components:

- assessment such as history taking or physical assessment
- planning of nursing care from a history or test result
- implementation of care including patient/staff education or nursing care.

Each situation must be designed to be completed within an identified time period, eg. ten minutes. Nicol and Freeth (1998) advise 25 minutes.

The situations can address the same competencies, such as history taking but the patient's condition will vary to allow the student to determine different information. Each situation must address a different aspect for assessemtn although there will be some overlap. The assessment forms may need to vary to allow for the differences in the patient's information.

These examples of situations that may be in a practical clinical assessment cover a range of conditions, including conditions applicable to different branches.

Situation 1: asks the student to take a nursing history from a patient who has recently had a myocardial infarction.

Situation 2: asks the student to give a patient discharge advice following a first myocardial infarction.

Situation 3: requires the student to take the blood pressure, both lying and standing, of a patient who has previously had a right sided cerebral vascular accident.

Situation 4: asks the student to take a history from a patient who is mentally disturbed.

Situation 5: asks the student to explain section 5(4) of the Mental Health Act to a nursing student on her first placement.

Situation 6: asks the student to inform a newly diagnosed active 18 year old on how to manage his epilepsy. Medication has been prescribed.

Situation 7: asks the student to take a history from a patient who has been admitted in a rather unkempt state.

Situation 8: asks the student to plan the care, with justification, for a patient who has been admitted in a rather unkempt state.

Situation 9: asks the student to explain the underlying theory of nursing and research that supports the plan of care for the patient who has been admitted in a rather unkempt state.

Situation 10: asks the student to teach a teenage patient and parent how to manage insulin injections.

Situation 11: asks the student to administer eye drops to a patient and advise him with regard to his discharge care.

Situation 12: asks the student to teach a patient/parent with regard to discharge information for steroid medication.

Activity 39

Consider a series of situations that could be linked to the learning experience of students and staff in your clinical area.

Each situation must consist of:

- an assessment scenario that is explained in writing
- relevant instruction with a set of marking criteria for the assessor.

An assessment scenario that is explained in writing

The following are examples of possible assessment scenarios.

Situation A

Mr Bones has arrived for admission to your clinical area complaining of headaches. Please take a relevant nursing history from this patient regarding his headaches.

Situation B

Mr F Jason has recently developed insulin dependent diabetes. He has been prescribed 36 units of insulin. He needs instruction with regard to the administration of his insulin injections.

Situation C

Mr E Simms has weakness of the upper limbs. He is able to sit unsupported on the edge of the bed but requires to be helped into the sitting position. Measure the blood pressure of Mr Simms in the lying and sitting positions. Record your findings on the sheet of plain paper and hand it to the examiner.

Activity 40

Select two areas of practice and discuss two situations which may be designed to assess a member of staff's knowledge, skills or attitudes.

Once a situation has been defined then the following are required for the assessor:

- relevant instructions
- marking criteria.

The following are three examples of possible instructions and marking criteria for the three previously mentioned situations.

Relevant instructions

Situation A

Instruction to assessor: observe the student conducting the assessment and do not interrupt. Place a tick in the appropriate area indicating that the student correctly covered the item. When there is no tick, it will be assumed that the student did not attempt to cover the item or did so incorrectly. Complete sections B and C by placing a circle around the appropriate comment.

Situation B

Instruction to assessor: Observe the student conducting the assessment and do not interrupt. Place a tick in the appropriate column for section a. Listen to the explanation and award a mark accordingly for section b.

Situation C

Instruction to assessor: Observe the student conducting the assessment and do not interrupt. Please tick the appropriate column indicating one of the following criteria: satisfactory; attempted and partly satisfactory; not attempted/unsatisfactory.

Marking criteria

Situation A

Mark sheet		Score 1 mark for each in section A	
A. History	**Score**		**Score**
1. onset		6. associated symptoms	
2. location		7. aggravating symptoms	
3. duration		8. relieving factors	
4. frequency		9. previous treatment	
5. characteristics		10. family history	
		Total A	

B. Overall technique

Assess whether systematic, prioritised and relevant:

Excellent	Good	Fair	Satisfactory	Unsatisfactory
5	4	3	2	1

Please circle one   **Total B**

C. Overall attitude toward patient

Assess consideration of patient's feelings, rapport:

Excellent	Good	Fair	Satisfactory	Unsatisfactory
5	4	3	2	1

Please circle one   **Total C**

Situation B

Assessment sheet (a)

	Indicate the following actions	Carried out satisfactorily	Attempted but not satisfactory
1	Checks prescription sheet		
2	Washes hands		
3	Withdraws appropriate units of air		
4	Swabs inuslin bottles		
5	Injects units of air into insulin		
6	Withdraws correct dose of insulin		
7	Checks total dose and eliminates air bubbles		
8	Checks insulin dose with trained staff		
9	Injects subcutaneously at 90 degree angle		
10	Correctly disposes of needle and syringe		

Assessment sheet (b)

Key points of explanation (b)	**Suggested mark**
Explains marking system of syringe	2
Explains different types of insulins	1
Explains need to inject air into bottles to prevent vacuum	1
Explains order of withdrawal and need to prevent cross-contamination of insulins	2
Explains where to inject insulin (thighs, abdomen and upper arms)	1
Reassures the patient throughout	2
Discusses psychological problems	1

Situation C
Measuring blood pressure

	Satisfactory	Attempted and partly satisfactory	Not attempted/ unsatisfactory
Explains procedure to patient			
Positions patient and clothing appropriately			
Secures cuff in correct position			
Locates brachial pulse			
Inflates cuff to suitable level (a) lying (b) sitting			
Releases cuff pressure slowly (a) lying (b) sitting			
Deflates cuff after each measurement			
Positions equipment safely throughout			
Assists patient			
Gentle and considerate			
Safe and efficient			
Leaves patient comfortable			
Shows awareness of patient comfort at end of procedure			
Records results			
Clearly and legibly			
Identifies lying and sitting blood pressures			

Activity 41

Design your own assessment tool to assess a member of staff in one of the following situations:
hand washing
admitting a patient to hospital
information given to a relative
drug administration
a situation of your choice (from *activity 40*).

Rationale for objective structured assessment:

- can be prearranged
- variables can be controlled
- prevents actual incident rehearsal
- allows for application of skills
- more reliable as same assessor for each situation
- allows for problems of assessment, eg. reliability to be sorted out prior to assessment
- can be anxiety provoking
- limits testing to a short or pre-determined period
- relies on good preparation and conduct of assessments
- tests several areas at one time
- does not require rehearsal (working with the assessor)
- allows assessor to observe only
- measures the actual practice therefore should measure standard of work on a continuous basis.

Activity 42

Look at the list of suggested assessment situations on *page 86*:

- examine the validity of the clinical assessment for a pre-registered nurse.

Consider whether some assessment situations are seen to be more relevant/valid for your particular area.

Activity 43

Select:

- a situation linked to the assessment of communication and write out the situation for the intended student
- design an assessment tool with guidance for the assessor — consider the rationale of your assessment tool.

(You have been provided with examples of assessment documents on *pages 88–90*.)

Interpretations of assessment results

Analysis of results

The assessment tools you have designed could be used as part of a controlled practical assessment situation.

Take for example the 12 situations mentioned earlier. Imagine these situations were used to assess 30 students.

Also, imagine that the students could be awarded a grade for each situation ranging from A to F. Grades A , B, C, D could be a pass while grades E and F could be a fail.

The results show an overall range of grades showing that:

Grade A was awarded on 38 occasions

Grade B on 56 occasions

Grade C on 90 occasions

Grade D on 100 occasions

Grade E on 36 occasions

Grade F on 40 occasions

Various interpretations of these results could be made. For example:

* There are 284 occasions when a student passed — this is derived from the total score of Grades A, B, C and D.

* There are 76 occasions when a student failed — the derived total score of Grades E and F.

These interpretations do not give the total number of students that passed or failed all the examination.

The pass rate of the total assessment situation in percentage terms is/could be 64%. This could appear to be a reasonable result overall, but there are many aspects to be considered as to whether this examination is valid and discriminatory.

The following are some aspects that may be considered to determine the assessment's validity and discriminatory ability:

Validity

- subject matter
- relevance of examination to teaching time or practical experience
- preparation of the students
- range of expectation

Discriminatory ability

- difficulty of some aspects of the examination

• ease of some aspects of the examination

Activity 44

Look at the set of results below, for the previously mentioned situations and determine as many reasons as possible for the results. Be guided by the considerations above. Remember there may be more than one reason for the good or poor results.

Table 4: Spread sheet of results of clinical examination

	30 students	A	B	C	D	E
1	History taking — myocardial infarction	6	10	7	7	
2	Discharge advice following myocardial infarction	4	9	8	9	
3	Taking a blood pressure	20	8	2		
4	History taking — mentally ill patient	3	2	19	4	2
5	Teaching — Mental Health Act	8	8	6	2	6
6	Teaching — condition and medication	4	14	10	2	
7	History taking — unknown condition	8	10	8	4	
8	Care planning	2	4	7	11	6
9	Theory and research linked to care	16	5	5	4	
10	Teaching — insulin injections	4	12	6	6	2
11	Discharge care, teaching — eye drops	4	6	17	3	
12	Teaching — discharge medication	3	10	14	3	
	Total scores	82	99	109	55	16

In looking at the results (*table 4*) it can be seen that some situations produce a better pass result. It could be concluded that these assessments are easy. However, other factors need to be considered.

The situation may require a definite action to produce safe practice and the results should not be anything but 100% satisfactory performance. In other words, good results need to be even better, eg. taking a blood pressure.

Some situations, eg. no 4 may mean that students' practical experience and its proximity to the examination may need to be questioned.

Other situations may mean that the students require further teaching or practical experience under supervision to attain these skills, eg. no 4.

Care planning in situation 8 appears to need further development;

however, the situation may need reviewing to ensure that the students have the necessary knowledge to complete the care planning.

Theory and research linked to patient care seems to be well learnt but is it too easy?

Situations 10, 11 and 12 appear to give a reasonable range of results to illustrate that the examination does discriminate. However, like all situations they still require an in-depth look at the itemised results of each student to determine if there are any internal inconsistencies.

Accreditation of prior experiential learning (APEL)

This is a fast developing form of assessment which uses relevant learning which has been acquired previously and applies it in a different context. For example, qualified nurses who have a wide range of clinical knowledge and experience, can demonstrate this learning in a written format.

Evidence presented for this type of assessment is normally within a profile whereby learning (usually in clinical practice) is recounted, reviewed and reflected upon in an academic format. Such profiles are assessed in order to gain academic credits (credit accumulation and transfer scheme — CATS) to gain entry either to a course or to be accredited with part of a course, ie. a module.

According to Simosko and Cook (1996) such profiles need to have the following hallmarks within the evidence submitted:

validity
reliability
sufficiency
authenticity
currency

The profile must be assessed against the learning outcomes for the module or against the admissions criteria, to ensure that **validity** is achieved.

Reliability is the responsibility of the assessor in that the module's learning outcomes or the criteria for admission are applied consistently to all candidates.

There should be **sufficient evidence** to equate to the volume or quality of work which would have been submitted by another student following a more traditional route. For example, if a student who was undertaking a module had to write an assignment of 2000 words at diploma level to gain 12 academic 'CATS' points, then a student submitting a profile should include a comparable amount of work written at diploma level. Academic rigour needs to be maintained. The person submitting the profile needs to ensure that the work is **verifiable** by others. The authentication can be in the form of awards such as certificates of achievement or attendance. However, the key element in a profile is the review and reflection on the learning which took place at the time and which has taken place since.

Each university will have its own regulations regarding AP(E)L assessment and there will be varying time limits given to the currency of the work submitted. Five years is the figure which is used in many institutions. Similarly, each university has its own process for dealing with accreditation of prior experiential learning. The individual applicant will need to adhere to the relevant process.

The type of profile discussed in this section is not the same as a UKCC personal professional profile required for re-registration but an expansion of similar principles.

The AP(E)L process is now well established and widely used in most universities. Many applicants for post-registration courses are finding that the AP(E)L process is enabling them to gain access to courses which were previously inaccessible. In a recent article Wilkinson (1998) concludes,

... this route to recognition of academic achievement is not easy *...*(but) *learning from experience is embedded in practice and so highly relevant to real life issues.*

Conclusion

At the end of this section the reader should be able to:
- identify four main types of assessment
- describe the advantages of each type of assessment identified
- present an objective structured clinical examination situation for own clinical area
- discuss bias and attitude towards assessees and/or patients
- be aware of the potential of AP(E)l process
- justify responses to the following situations:
  * Jessica asks that although she is being assessed by continuous assessment she could also have an arranged drug round assessment.
  * Danny has observed some medical students on the ward doing ward based objective structured examinations and

he asks why this cannot be arranged for him and the other students in the clinical area.

References and suggested further reading

Bradshaw PL (ed) (1989) *Teaching and Assessing in Clinical Nursing Practice.* Prentice Hall, London

Brown RA, Hawksley B (1996) *Learning Skills, Studying Styles and Profiling.* Quay Books, Mark Allen Publishing Group, Salisbury

Bujack L, McMillan M, Dwyer J *et al* (1991) Assessing comprehensive nursing performance: the objective structural clinical assessment (OSCA) Part 1 — Development of the assessment strategy. *Nurse Ed Today* **11**: 179–184

Bujack L, McMillan M, Dwyer J *et al* (1991) Assessing comprehensive nursing performance: the objective structural clinical assessment (OSCA) Part 2 — Report of the evaluation project. *Nurse Ed Today* **11**: 248–255

Clifford C (1994) Assessment of clinical practice and the role of the nurse teacher. *Nurse Ed Today* **14**: 272–279

Everden JJ (1986) Preparing for change: an investigation into the attitudes of assessors to ward-based assessments as a preliminary to continuing clinical assessments. *J Adv Nurs* **11**: 713–718

Everett A (1995) The educational role of the community mental health nurse. *Ment Health Nurs* **15**(9): 8–10

Exton, Smith (1976) Management of ward-based assessments. Cited in: Everden JJ (1986) Preparing for change: an investigation into the attitudes of assessors to ward-based assessments as a preliminary to continuing clinical assessments. *J Adv Nurs* **11**: 713–718

Ghaye A, Lillyman S (1997) *Learning Journals and Critical Incidents: reflective practice for health care professionals.* Quay Books, Mark Allen Publishing Group, Salisbury

Girot EA (1993) Assessment of competence in clinical practice — a review of the literature. *Nurse Ed Today* **13**: 83–90

Kenworthy N, Nicklin P (1989) *Teaching and Assessing in Nursing Practice. An experiential approach.* Scutari, London

Lillyman S, Evans B (1996) *Designing a Portfolio/Profile. A Workbook for Health Care Professionals.* Quay Books, Mark Allen Publishing Group, Salisbury

MacGuire J (1984) Assessing the assessor. *Senior Nurse* **9**(1): 12–13

Nicol M, Freeth D (1998) Assessment of clinical skills: a new approach to an old problem. *Nurse Ed Today* **18**: 601–609

Oldfield S (1996) Case studies of good practice. *New Academic* **5**(1): 10–11

Oppenheim AN (1984) *Questionnaire Design and Attitude Measurement.* Heinemann, London

Ross M, Carroll G, Knight J *et al* (1988) Using the OSCE to measure clinical skills performance in nursing. *J Adv Nurs* **13**: 45–56

Schon DA (1983) *The reflective practitioner: how professionals think in action.* Temple Smith, London

Simosko S, Cook C (1996) *Applying APL Principles in Flexible Assessment: A Practical Guide,* 2nd edn. Kogan Page, London

Stoker D, Hull C (1994) Assessment in learning ii) Assessment and learning outcomes. *Nurs Times* (Open Learning Supplement) **90**(12): ii–vii

UKCC (1996) *Position Statement on Clinical Supervision for Nurses, Midwives and Health Visitors.* UKCC, London

Wilkinson J (1998) Academic accreditation. *Nurs Standard* **3**(7): 42–44

8
Assessment of teaching

It is not only the practice of nursing that needs to be assessed but aspects related to the nurse's role of a health promoter and educator. This aspect can often involve teaching patients, relatives or other members of staff. The teaching session itself can become the focus of the assessment situation.

This chapter will look at the assessment of a teaching session. The assessment of teaching is often prearranged — that is the teacher to be assessed will be made aware that s/he is going to be assessed. There is a possibility that a definitive time period has not been determined but a fact that the assessment will occur within a set number of weeks. In these situations it is worth considering whether the assessee is told definitely in advance so that he/she can decide on subsequent action for the learner/s to be involved in the teaching situation.

The influence of a 'stranger' (assessor) in the teaching situation may disturb the learner. If the learner is not told about the assessment situation they may feel curious about the 'stranger'.

If the learner is told about the assessment situation s/he may respond contrary to normal by being either very positive or equally negative and obstructive to the assessee.

See section on patient selection in *chapter 6*.

In arranging the assessment the assessor must ensure that the assessee is shown the requirements of the assessment. An assessment tool is needed.

Activity 45

> In order to compile an assessment tool, list the component parts of a teaching session.

The component parts of a teaching session can form the aspects to be examined in the assessment session. These can be looked at and derived from the stages of the nursing process: assessment /planning / implementation/evaluation.

The considerations for a teaching session involve:

* **Assessment** of the teaching session and the environment:
    Topic
    Learner entry knowledge

Expected learning from teaching session
Time both in the day/week and the duration
Environment and available visual aids.

* **Planning** to achieve the identified aim and objectives of the teaching session. This means that consideration needs to be given to the following:

    Relevance of session to the learner — the more immediate or important creates attention and enhances learning.

    Motivational aids (see section on motivation *chapter 2*).

    Memory — a limited capacity exists in most minds but this can be improved by repeating important points.

    Sequence — correct sequence and logical arrangement of information will aid retention. Working from known to unknown also helps memory.

    Strategy — means considering the most appropriate teaching method/methods to convey the information. This may mean a lecture, a question and answer session or a demonstration.

* **Implementation** /delivery of the session as planned or as adapted to the situation which presents, eg. curtailing length of session due to unexpected events in the clinical area. Also included is the student interaction.

* **Evaluation** of the effectiveness of the session, which can mean incorporating into the session learner/assessee self-assessment.

This evaluation could involve learner:

* responding in praise/criticism
* correctly answering questions

The evaluation could also involve the assessee's:

* appropriate clarification of points or questions
* response to whether the session would be done again in the same way.

It can also mean reviewing the objectives of the teaching session to assess the learning that has occurred.

The following tool looks at the assessment of a teaching session. The aspects to be looked for occur on the left hand of the page and the level is indicated as satisfactory/or needs improvement.

	Satisfactory	Needs improvement
Introduction of self		
Introduction of session		
Aim written and stated correctly		
Objectives written and stated correctly		
Awareness of students' entry behaviour		
Preparation of environment		
Sequence of session — content — organisation		
Use of visual aids		
Interaction with students		
Use of language and voice		
Conclusion — assessment of learning		
Timing		

Although this form outlines the aspects to be looked for it does not give a great deal of detail as to the level required.

For example, what is satisfactory about timing?

If you are doing a 30 minute teaching session should the timing be exact or could it be like a theoretical assessment: an assignment that can be 10% either way of the word limit. In the case of this teaching assessment, could it be 27 or 33 minutes and still be satisfactory?

Alternative assessment tools may look at other aspects and not necessarily at the time period.

Two aspects that link to timing have been selected from an assessment tool.

delivery	speaks much too fast	too quick	about right	too slow	tediously slow
material	far too much	rather too much	satisfac-tory	rather too little	too little content

This assessment tool has given five different choices to be made concerning speed of delivery and amount of material. The more choices there are possible the more chance of covering every option, but is there a clear distinction between the statements to allow for reliability? For example, what is the exact difference between rather too much/satisfactory/rather too little?

Some assessment tools give a choice of five decisions ranging from a good statement to a poor statement, eg.

	1	2	3	4	5	
Speaks much too fast						Tediously slow

Other assessment tools leave the assessor with a space for individual comment (possibly subjective comment) guided only by an overall statement.

Activity 46

Comment on outline of session, logical timing sequence, relevance of content.

Activity 47

Design your own assessment tool to assess a teaching session.

Conclusion

At the end of this section the reader should be able to:

- devise an assessment tool to assess a teaching session.
- assess a teaching session
- give appropriate feedback following the assessment of a teaching session in the clinical area
- consider responses to the following situations:

  * both Jessica and Danny are in a teaching session led by an ENB course 998 student. Jessica's opinion is that even though it meant she was late off duty the session was so good it was worth it. Danny said it was all too theoretical for a ward based teaching session. As the official assessor of the teaching session how would you evaluate the session using the student's responses as evidence?

  * you are officially assessing a member of staff teaching Danny and Jessica and you note that the assessee has given the students some incorrect information concerning the location of the equipment they are referring to. What action would you take?

References and suggested further reading

Bradshaw PL (ed) (1989) *Teaching and Assessing in Clinical Nursing Practice*. Prentice Hall, London

Child D (1986) *Psychology and the Teacher,* 4th edn. Cassell Education, London

Cotton J (1995)*The Theory of Assessment — An Introduction.* Kogan Page, London

Kenworthy N, Nicklin P (1989) *Teaching and Assessing in Nursing Practice. An experiential approach.* Scutari, London

Quinn FM (1995) *Principles and Practice of Nurse Education*, 3rd edn. Chapman Hall, London

Rowntree D (1987) *Assessing Students: How shall we know them?* Kogan Page, London

Appendix

Rule 18a

The stated professional competencies in Nursing, Midwifery and Health Visitors Rules Approved Order 1989, No 1456 (September, 1989).

a. The identification of the social and health implications of pregnancy and child bearing, physical and mental handicap, disease, disability, or ageing for the individual, her or his friends, family and community.

b. The recognition of common factors which contribute to, and those which adversely affect, physical, mental and social well-being of patients and clients and take appropriate action.

c. The use of relevant literature and research to inform the practice of nursing.

d. The appreciation of the influence of social, political and cultural factors in relation to health care.

e. An understanding of the requirements of legislation relevant to the practice of nursing.

f. The use of appropriate communication skills to enable the development of helpful caring relationships with patients and clients and their families and friends, and to initiate and conduct relationships with patients and clients.

g. The identification of health related learning needs of patients and clients, families and friends and to participate in health promotion.

h. An understanding of the ethics of health care and of the nursing profession and the responsibility which these impose on the nurse's professional practice.

i. The identification of the needs of patients and clients to enable them to progress from varying degrees of dependence to maximum independence, or to a peaceful death.

j. The identification of physical, psychological, social and spritual needs of the patients or client; and awareness of values and concepts of individual care; the ability to devise a plan of care, contribute to its implementation and evaluation; and the demonstration of a problem-solving approach to the care of patients and clients.

k. The ability to function effectively in a team and participate in a multi-professional approach to the care of patients and clients.

l. The use of the appropriate channel of referral for matters not within her sphere of competence.

m. The assignment of appropriate duties to others and the supervision, teaching and monitoring of assigned duties.

Index